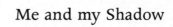

Me and my Shadow

Me and my Shadow

Learning to live with
Multiple Sclerosis

CAROLE MACKIE

WITH SUE BRATTLE

Aurum Press

In memory of Ronnie Lane

In admiration of his efforts to create
awareness of multiple sclerosis.
His determination to find a cure was
inspiring. For everyone in the world
who has MS, I pray that one day
we will find a cure.

First published in Great Britain 1999
by Aurum Press Ltd
25 Bedford Avenue, London WC1B 3AT

Text copyright © 1999 by Sue Brattle and Carole Mackie

A catalogue record for this book is available from
the British Library.

ISBN 1 85410 627 9

1 3 5 7 9 10 8 6 4 2
1999   2001   2003   2002   2000

Typeset by York House Typographic, London
Printed in Great Britain by MPG Books, Bodmin

CONTENTS

Foreword

I am delighted that Carole Mackie has dedicated this book to the memory of Ronnie Lane. Our days together in the Faces were some of the most exciting and memorable times of my life. It was a tragedy when Ronnie was struck down with MS and he battled bravely with the illness for more than twenty years. His contribution to music was finally recognised with a prestigious Ivor Novello award in the year prior to his death.

I wish Carole every success with the book and have the greatest admiration for all her efforts to raise public awareness of MS.

RONNIE WOOD

ACKNOWLEDGEMENTS

I would like to thank the following people. My mother: you are my inspiration. I love you. My father for being there. I love you, dad. Hazel for her love and support. All my wonderful friends; knowing you're there gives me strength. Craig and Maggie whose honesty has been invaluable.

British Airways, cabin crew, Scheduling, Community Relations, Dr Mooney and Dr Bagshaw for allowing some normality in my life. Dr Worthington and all at The Rowans Surgery for their patience and understanding. David, Adrian, Peter, Ken and Ruth for your support, encouragement, guidance and dedication. Claire, Barbara and Trish at Merton MS Society — what would I do without you? Nick Cowan, Jamie and Steve for their help in making things happen.

Ronnie Wood and Rod Stewart for their involvement and support. Thanks to Trebletrim Limited for a photograph of Ronnie Wood. Carlton at New Millennium Communications for caring. Colin and Maxine for their practical guidance, time and support. Sue Brattle who believed in me every step of the way and whose time, talent, dedication and invaluable guidance gave me strength. Finally, Sheila Murphy for making our dream become a reality.

1. A Trip to Rio

Bliss! I snuggled down on the sofa with Craig, glancing at my watch. Seven o'clock. I might just manage to have the quiet night in that I needed. We had precious little spare time, so even after two years together it was still a novelty to have an evening at home, just the two of us.

'Do you think it's safe to start cooking?' asked Craig. He was so sweet as he pampered me after a third bout of sinusitis – not the most attractive of illnesses. His job as a golf professional and mine as an air stewardess kept us apart for most of the year, so I hated it if I was ill when we were together. It seemed such a waste of time. That's when the phone rang. Damn!

'It's for you,' Craig said, passing the phone over to me, getting all the wires wrapped up around us and making me giggle.

'Hello Carole, it's British Airways, we have a flight for you.' My heart sank as I saw my evening slip away from me. Being on standby didn't happen often and this was the worst bit of it, planning an evening in your head then having it ruined.

'It's a 10-day trip, Rio de Janeiro.' I sat bolt upright on the edge of the sofa. 'Is everything OK, Caz, what's the matter?' Craig asked. What should I do? If I looked too excited it would hurt his feelings, but this was the one trip I'd been after for months. I'd been a long-haul stewardess for two years and had never managed to make it to Rio. Now, here it was. I put down the phone and told him. His face dropped slightly, but this was how we lived. It would be my turn to pull long faces next month, when he was off to Finland for another six-month stay as the pro at a golf club outside Helsinki.

I had four hours before the flight. I went into the bedroom and put on my uniform, picked up my suitcase (shorts, T-shirts, jeans, dress, swimming costume, sun cream, always packed) and went out into the living-room to say goodbye to Craig. He always said there was a nice balance between our jobs, that it kept the relationship healthy. At that moment, though, I wanted to stay with him.

'Oh Craig, I really don't want to go.'

'Never mind, Caz, it's only 10 days,' he said. 'Then we'll have a nice time together before I go away.'

'I'll send you a postcard from Copacabana Beach!'

'You lucky thing.' We had one last hug and I left.

I enjoyed the drive from my flat in Streatham across London to Heathrow Airport. You couldn't describe it as pretty with streets and streets of red-brick terraced houses all looking the same. But it was time to myself in my pride and joy, my lovely white Jeep. It always cheered me up. As I was sitting at red traffic lights about a mile from our flat it struck me how lucky I was. I still hadn't lost the thrill of seeing a new country, yet I had Craig to come home to. I smiled. Who'd have guessed from our first encounter that we'd still be going strong? We met at the cash and carry warehouse where his brother was the manager. How romantic! Craig happened to be there one day when I'd gone along to buy shampoo and stuff like that.

By 10 o'clock Heathrow was buzzing. My flight to Rio was packed. I was fighting to keep awake, let alone prepare for 10 hours in the air. But it's a funny thing with flying, however tired or grumpy you feel on the ground, the job sort of takes over once you're on the move. It's like putting on a performance, you make the effort to be bright and breezy.

That's what I was doing as I served the passengers on the upper deck. I was trained for Boeing 747s, Jumbo jets, what I call real aeroplanes, and I love them. The plane was soon quiet and peaceful, as it always is on overnight flights. The purser and I sat in the galley munching chocolate and drinking coffee to keep ourselves awake. It's unhealthy, but it works and you never know when a passenger is going to need you.

We all took turns to snatch some sleep in a crew bunk in the tail of the plane but I was awake and had put on fresh make-up before it was time to see to the breakfasts. As I was topping up the coffee cups, it dawned on me that this was a 10-day stay, so I'd be able to do all the sightseeing I wanted. We had one shuttle flight to do, to Sao Paolo, but other than that our time was our own. I could top up my tan as well as going up Sugar Loaf Mountain. For once I'd be able to tick everything off my list instead of cramming too much into a few hours. This crew were a nice crowd, too, with a few old faces I hadn't seen for ages. There'd be a lot of catching up to do.

The captain sounded the three chimes, the signal for the cabin crew to sit down and strap themselves in for landing. I looked out of a window and caught my first glimpse of the huge statue of Christ The Redeemer standing on the mountain top. Rio sprawled across hills and down to the sea for miles and miles around.

We already knew the weather was perfect; blue, cloudless skies and temperatures of 90 degrees and more. After we landed and the cabin door was opened a blast of heat hit me. It was a moment I loved at the end of any flight but this time it was special. I was 23 years old and in Rio, the city at the top of my wish-list when I'd decided to become a stewardess.

The crew's job is over once all the passengers are off the plane, so we all clambered straight onto the bus and headed for our hotel. As usual I sat on the back seat and opened a window to have a cigarette. I put my Walkman on and prepared to soak up the sights.

'Hey, Carole, are you on for a gin and tonic by the pool?' one of the stewardesses shouted over my tape of Lionel Richie.

'OK,' I said, 'but I want a swim as well. This heat's amazing.'

The bus was tearing along a wide, busy main road. Suddenly, as I lay sprawled across the seat, I felt really sleepy. Through half-closed eyes I realized I was looking at hundreds of thin, nut-brown women promenading along the one stretch of sand I'd always wanted to sunbathe on – Copacabana Beach.

'I didn't know you could fit that many bodies on to one beach,' I wailed. In London I'd thought my light tan looked good; here I just looked washed out. I thought of Craig back home.

'White sand, blue sky and naked girls on the beach,' had been his answer when I'd asked him ages ago what he thought Rio would be like. He was spot on.

I was just thinking I'd buy him a postcard and tell him how right he was when the change hit me; it had taken only a few minutes but suddenly we were out of the posh bit and right in the middle of a shanty town. A group of little children sat on the dusty roadside holding out their hands for money. Their mothers pulled them back as our bus sped by, the dirt and dust in our wake floating into the open doors of their corrugated iron huts.

The women looked about the same age as me. It made me think; I was so lucky, with everything to look forward to. What on earth forced them out of bed every morning, struggling to survive each day and never knowing what the future held? Our lives couldn't be more different. Just as suddenly the squalor was behind us. The bus climbed up and up a steep and winding hill, and there was the Rio Sheraton, home for the trip.

Cabin crew always have the energy for a first drink when they arrive anywhere. It didn't matter that I'd barely slept for a day. I went up to my room, climbed out of my uniform and into T-shirt and shorts, and was back in the lobby in 15 minutes. We gathered round the pool, a slight breeze blowing in off the beach spread out below us, chatting, arranging the evening and soaking up the sunshine. I'd left a grey and wet March in England. Just a few minutes with a drink in one hand, a cigarette in the other and the sun beating down on me and I felt great. This was heaven!

One by one we went to our rooms as the need for sleep caught up with us. I took the lift to the fifteenth floor, went into my room and grabbed a bottle of mineral water from the mini-bar. I clicked the lock on the huge window that ran down one side of the room, slid it open and stepped out onto my tiny balcony. Sitting in my own little world, I could just hear the muffled sound of tennis balls being hit on the courts below. But my eyes were drawn to the statue of Christ. I had seen so many pictures of it and here it was, so familiar and so powerful. I had a perfect view of it and it would be all mine for 10 days. Much as I loved my little flat in London, its view of the residents' car park just couldn't compare.

I must have slept all afternoon because when I woke up it was dark outside and the hotel was quiet. I felt fuzzy and it took a few seconds for me to remember where I was. I rolled over in my huge double bed and looked at my little alarm clock. I had three-quarters of an hour to shower and dress. Four of us were meeting at eight o'clock in the lobby to go out for a bite to eat.

I took a slow shower and sat down at the dressing table to put on my make-up. That shower was the last thing I did in what I now think of as my old life. Then something happened that was going to change me, my life, everything, for ever.

I squeezed a drop of moisturiser onto my fingers and started to rub it gently into my face. I couldn't feel anything. My fingertips had gone completely numb.

I realized how tired I must be; flying throws out your body clock and I was used to having aches and pains at odd times. That must be it. So I finished my make-up and started to dress.

I did up my bra, back to front as usual so I could see the hooks and eyes. As I twisted it round the right way, with the fastening at the back, I couldn't feel anything. Normally, there'd be a slight sensation as the bra rubbed against my ribcage, but this time, nothing. I had a band about two inches deep around my chest that was numb.

What was going on?

It seems unbelievable now, looking back, but I didn't really give any of this a second thought. I raced along the corridor, down to the lobby, and four of us went out on the town. Mind you, we were back by 11 and I slept like a log. We'd passed dozens of nightclubs, but we knew we had lots of time here so there was no rush. We'd go clubbing when we all felt a bit more awake.

The next morning my holiday began. I was in the mood for it, too. The tiredness had gone, the sun was blazing down, and the pool looked cool and tempting. There were already people lazing on the sun loungers and I wanted to be one of them, but I'd have breakfast first. I put on a T-shirt and a pair of leggings. As I pulled the leggings up I couldn't feel my waistline. I knew that the elastic on their waistband was rubbing my skin because it was making a little mark, but I couldn't feel it. Perhaps it was time I mentioned this to someone.

After breakfast I popped back up to my room and put on my swimming costume under a pair of shorts and a T-shirt. I made my way down to the pool where some of the crew were already settled in. I took off my shorts and sat on the edge of a lounger while I pulled my T-shirt over my head. A stewardess called Annette was on the lounger next to mine and I put my book and suntan cream, pen, post-cards and stamps on the little white table between us. This was our first flight together so we didn't know each other, but that's crew life. You make friends within hours when you're flying with someone, and then don't see them for months or even years.

Annette is as dark-haired, dark-eyed and olive-skinned as I am blonde, blue-eyed and fair-skinned. I envied her as she made herself comfortable, a bikini and Factor 2 all she needed between her skin and the sun. I reckoned I'd have 15 minutes without my T-shirt on, then cover up for my first day. It was no good ruining everything with sunburn.

'I've got no feeling around my waist,' I said to her as I lay back on the lounger. 'It's really weird. I can't explain it.'

'Do you think you should tell the doctor, Carole?' Her Manchester accent conjured up rain rather than Rio.

'No, I won't bother him,' I said. 'I probably just slept awkwardly. It'll go away. Strange, though.'

I put on my sunglasses. The sky looked purple through the lenses and the heat scorched into my skin, making me feel relaxed and lazy. I stretched out. This was perfect. There was one thing missing, of course. Craig. I knew he'd love it here and it was such a romantic setting. What a waste! I wrote him a postcard: 'Everything's perfect but I wish you were here'. It felt like it was going to be ages before I saw him again. I went into the hotel lobby, everything turning dark suddenly as I came out of the sun, and posted the card. Then it was time for a gin and tonic and lunch. What a life – and I was being paid for it.

We all agreed to spend the rest of the day around the pool. It looked irresistible with its little bridge across from the sunbathing area to the bar. We could do some showing-off later as the diving board end was overlooked by a glass-walled restaurant. Someone pointed out that even in Rio it's not sunny all the time, so we should make the most of it. If the clouds rolled down from the mountains above us, that would be the time for some sightseeing, so I decided to go for a swim. I'd already had a morning doing nothing and I had no intention of letting my exercise programme slip, holiday or no holiday.

I started to climb the ladder down the side of the pool at the deep end. Other crew members who were already swimming shouted that the water was warm. It covered my ankles, then my knees and my thighs. I looked down and could see my feet gripping onto the ladder's rungs, splayed out and distorted under the water.

But I couldn't feel a thing.

I kept climbing down. The water came up to my waist, then my hands were submerged and my arms. Still no feeling. At last, as the water lapped over my shoulders, I had a sensation of wet warmth.

I slid off the ladder and trod water. I must have bobbed up and down for 10 minutes, not saying a word, letting everyone forget I was there. I couldn't feel anything from just beneath my shoulders down to my toes, and yet everything was normal from the shoulders up. I didn't understand what was happening. I wasn't scared but I didn't quite know what to do.

I swam over to the side of the pool and lifted myself up to the edge, sitting for a few more minutes with just my feet in the water. I splashed about, one foot in front of the other, a flash of pink nail polish as my toes came out of the water then disappeared back under again. I knew I was doing it because I could see it. But I couldn't feel a thing. It was time to call the doctor but first things first; I needed a drink. I walked over to the raffia-roofed bar by the poolside and a Brazilian in a spotless white jacket poured me a gin and tonic. I took it back to where the crew were sitting.

'Enjoy your swim, Carole? You looked very restful out there.' My purser from the flight out smiled as I sat down and lit a cigarette.

'I couldn't feel the water,' I said, quietly and slowly. 'I think I've been bitten by something. Or I've picked up a virus. What do you think? I couldn't feel anything.' I was drying myself with a hotel towel as I spoke and looked up to see a frown on the purser's face. Only a few hours ago he and I had been whispering gossip to each other as our passengers slept on the upper deck.

'I think I should tell the captain,' he said. 'Let's get the doctor to look at you. It's probably nothing but it's best to check. Will you meet me in the lobby when you're dressed? Don't rush, Carole.'

By the time I'd finished my drink and wandered into the air-conditioned cool of the hotel the purser was standing by the reception desk chatting to a dark-haired man in glasses. I shivered as the heat from outdoors melted away.

'My name is Dr Fritz,' he said as I came up to them. He shook my hand. 'I'm surprised you're still walking, Carole.'

He wanted to give me a proper examination. Annette and two more of the crew insisted on coming up to my room with me. It was odd, I did feel a bit unsure on my feet. But I wasn't worried – just annoyed that this was going to eat into our sunbathing time.

'OK everyone, sorry about this. But the mini bar's on me!' I said as we all made our way up to the fifteenth floor. Dr Fritz raised his eyebrows slightly. Poor man! But he was the BA doctor here in Rio so he was used to cabin crew.

We reached my room and I cleared all the clutter off the bed and sofa. I opened the long window and poured everyone, except me and the doctor, a drink. They all sat down. Dr Fritz asked me to lie on the bed on my stomach and he explained he was going to use a tiny pin to test my reactions.

I lay there for ages, staring into my pillow and wishing he'd get on with it, but nothing happened. Then I felt a tiny pinprick. 'Ouch,' I shouted as the pin went into the flesh on my right shoulder. One of the crew laughed but as I rolled over I saw a look of concern pass between Annette and one of the other girls.

'Now I am going to embarrass you in front of everyone,' the doctor said to me. 'I want you to pull faces at me, open your mouth as wide as it will go and stick out your tongue.'

He was right, I was embarrassed, but I was glad the crew were there. I wasn't too concerned but I didn't understand why the numbness seemed to be spreading. Next Dr Fritz asked me to walk a straight line, along the pattern in the carpet which stretched between my bed and the bathroom door.

'If you don't mind, Carole, I'd like another opinion,' he said. 'I want to ask a neurologist friend of mine to take a look at you. It won't take long to get him over here.' He walked over to the phone as Annette took me by the arm.

'We think you should know, Carole,' she said looking serious, 'but the doctor was sticking that pin into you for ages before you reacted. He'd put it in the soles of your feet, up the backs of your legs, and up your back.'

'I bet I've been bitten,' I said. Dr Fritz called me over. The neurologist arrived within minutes. He had been out on a call near the hotel so had reached us in double quick time. I went through all the same tests again. He told me I'd have to go into hospital.

'No, I don't want to,' I said. 'If there's something so wrong with me that I need a hospital why can't I go home?'

We called the captain up to my room and he asked the neurologist the same question. His answer made me realize I should take all this more seriously.

'You can fly her home,' he told the captain, 'as long as you carry a life support machine on board and are prepared to divert for landing at any time. We don't know what's wrong with Carole so we can't let you put her in any danger.'

The room went silent as everyone looked at me. I did what I always do when I'm really nervous: I laughed out loud. I lit a cigarette and Dr Fritz managed a disapproving look before ringing his wife to say he'd be home late. She didn't believe him!

'All she can hear is girls' voices and laughing,' he said when he came off the phone. 'She thinks I'm at a party.'

The crew were looking anxious but my only instinct was to phone

Craig. I wasn't too worried for myself but I didn't want him to phone the hotel and have a receptionist telling him that I was in hospital. It would be better for it to come from me.

'Craig Mitchell on the line for you,' the telephonist said as I waited for my call to England.

'All right, Cazzy Mac, what's happening?' The familiar Scottish accent with just a trace of concern in it made me determined to keep this conversation light and casual.

'Hi, Craig. I'm just ringing to let you know that I've got to go into hospital here for a few tests. I've gone a bit numb. It's nothing to worry about, though. I feel fine.'

'You're sure? OK, Caz. Give me a call when you know more. Love you.'

'I'll stay with you, Carole,' Annette said when I came off the phone. 'Someone had better make sure they don't do anything they shouldn't!' Everyone laughed, including me. It lightened the mood in the room as I packed an overnight bag.

A hotel car took Annette and me back down the winding hill we'd come up in the coach the day before and into the back streets of Rio. It was a short journey, the streets quiet in the afternoon heat. We drew up outside an ordinary looking building, more like an apartment block than a hospital.

I felt a bit of a fraud as we settled into the waiting room. An American woman who'd just gone into labour was there and as Annette and I chatted with her I honestly forgot what was happening to me. Annette can talk the hind legs off a donkey and I was glad she was with me as we laughed and joked with the mum-to-be.

The hospital wasn't a bit clinical. It smelt of polish rather than illness. The wooden floors and furniture made it seem more like a suite of offices, really. After a while Annette and I were taken up to my room on the second floor. One single iron bed, one sofa, and the bathroom and shower across the corridor. The air conditioning unit seemed to be broken and the room was stifling. I longed to be back at the Sheraton.

I threw open a window and looked down on a busy side street. The sound of cars and motorbikes revving their engines at a set of traffic lights just along from the hospital was deafening. I tried the air conditioning instead. It spluttered into life, then made such a racket I decided to stick with the open window and street sounds. At least it was contact with the outside world.

By the next night my breezy 'I feel fine' to Craig seemed a lifetime away. I just wanted him with me. Annette and I had locked our door for that first night in the hospital, though I don't know what we were afraid of. I think it was more a sign of how edgy we both felt. Poor Annette. She was automatically saying: 'I'm English,' to everyone who came into the room now. Her dark colouring made all the staff assume she was Brazilian and could speak Portuguese.

Our day had started with a vengeance, the first nurse coming in for a blood sample from me at 5.30 a.m. As the day wore on, I became more and more worried. At lunchtime I'd been tempted to use a spoon rather than a knife and fork to scoop up the chicken casserole, but I'd persevered. My fingers felt as if they belonged to someone else, that they weren't connected to my brain at all. My hands lay in my lap almost lifeless when I wasn't making an effort to use them. It was tiring to keep them rigid rather than let them just flop down from the wrists. My legs felt heavy, too. When we heard that the American woman's baby had been born I was shocked at what a struggle it was for me to walk along to her room. It was only a few steps down the corridor. Coming back I'd had to lean on Annette.

By the time I was having a second set of X-rays in the afternoon and the doctor asked me to raise my arms above my head, the weakness made me feel scared. It was becoming real. Craig had rung my dad in Devon to tell him what was happening. He had told my sister, Hazel, and she'd told our mum. They all rang the hospital to see if I was OK and asked if I wanted them with me. But the truth was that I only wanted Craig. I couldn't ask my mum without asking my dad, and it would have been their first meeting since their divorce. I certainly didn't want that meeting to be at my bedside! It was all too complicated and far too emotional for me to cope with right now.

Dr Fritz popped in to warn me that I'd need a lumbar puncture.

'What on earth's that?'

'They just need some fluid from your spine for tests,' he'd said.

It sounded disgusting, but I'd had so many tests by then that one more seemed neither here nor there.

Two nurses came in to my room first thing the next morning, chatting away in Portuguese. One gestured for me to lie in the foetal position with my legs curled up. Annette said one had a huge needle.

'Can you watch everything really closely so you can tell me what's going on?' I asked her. Then I felt a needle go into my back, at the base of my spine, and come out again just as quickly.

'That's not the big needle, Carole,' Annette said from the edge of the bed. 'I think that's just the anaesthetic.'

'Thank God for that. At least I won't be able to feel the real thing!'

Then I felt the big needle start to go in. The pain made me feel sick. It was a red-hot sensation that made my ears fizz, as though I was about to pass out. I wanted to cry and cry but couldn't because the needle was still in and I couldn't move. One nurse had his arms around me, holding me in position. He was trying to say something to me, but we didn't understand each other. I wanted to get up off the bed and run away. This couldn't be happening!

When the nurses had gone I forced myself into the bathroom so I could sit down and cry. It was cooler in there. I ran the tap in the sink to drown out my whimpering. I didn't want to worry Annette. I just stared at the white tiles, not quite believing the situation I was in. I was beginning to feel scared now and I didn't know what the lumbar puncture had done to me. Surely nothing should hurt that much?

I struggled back to bed and lay down on my side – my back was too sore to lie on – then drifted into sleep. When I woke up a little while later and lifted my head it hurt so much that I cried out.

'Annette, I can't bear this, I can't!' We pressed the panic button and a nurse came in almost immediately. She took one look at me and held my face firmly in both her hands, whispering soothing words. I wept. 'Dr Fritz, please, Dr Fritz.' I looked at her and she understood.

He was with me in less than 20 minutes, shocked and angry that I'd been moving about after the lumbar puncture.

'You must keep absolutely still,' he said. 'Don't move, don't move at all. They have drained some of the protective fluid from around your spine. Every movement will hurt and you could do some damage to yourself.'

I realized too late that the nurse had been trying to tell me to keep my head still.

I slept on and off for the rest of that day, vaguely aware that Annette was there, on the sofa, flicking through magazines, reading her book, or just staring out of the window. As the day wore on the sun disappeared, leaving a grey sky and humid heat that seemed to suck the energy from everyone. Even the nurses walked slowly. When Annette came back from a stroll down the road strands of her hair stuck to her damp face.

A few minutes later the rain came down, bouncing off the pavements below and forcing us to close our window. Good, we thought, perhaps it won't be so hot. But the clattering air conditioning unit and ceiling fan couldn't cool us down. I felt so tired and so scared that the simplest blood test that afternoon made me weepy with the pain of yet another needle going into my arm.

I needed Craig with me, he'd make things better. He had rung to say BA was trying to get him onto a flight to Rio but I'd heard nothing since. The thought of his smile made me cry into my pillow. What was happening to me? I didn't feel in control of what was going on. I wanted Craig to take control of everything for me. He'd have laughed if I'd told him that, but it made me realize how much the past few days had taken out of me.

I felt really ill when I was woken up at the crack of dawn for yet another blood test. Annette looked washed out, too. Three nights on an uncomfortable sofa were beginning to show.

'Annette, go back to the hotel later on and have a break,' I said to her. 'You'll go stir crazy stuck here with me.'

As soon as she had gone, after promising to come back that evening and bring along other crew to visit me, I gave Craig a ring. I half hoped he wouldn't answer, that he was already flying to me and had decided to surprise me by turning up out of the blue. But the phone only rang once before it was picked up, as though he was sitting next to it. I could feel hysteria creeping into my voice. The time for staying calm had passed.

'There's a bit of a delay, Carole,' he said, gently. 'They can't find a flight for me just yet.' Oh no, don't say he's not going to get here. I started to cry, the one thing I hadn't wanted to do.

'Please get here as soon as you can, Craig. I'm starting to get scared.'

I put down the phone and sobbed, my head in my hands. Just then Dr Fritz walked through the door. He stood still for a moment, horrified.

'My God, Carole, what's happened?' he asked, rushing across my room to my bed.

I told him everything in a jumble, gabbling about the lumbar puncture and Craig, how I was finding it difficult to use a knife and fork, my legs feeling like dead weights and how tired and weak I was.

'I'll see what I can do.'

Dr Fritz faxed Heathrow Airport from the hospital's administration office. He told BA that my situation was deteriorating and that Craig should be flown out to me as soon as possible. He came back up to my room when the fax had been sent. Dr Fritz, my saviour! I felt calmer once I knew somebody had done something. After he'd left I locked my door and slept.

The pain from the lumbar puncture was beginning to ease by the next morning. I could move my head properly without feeling as though huge metal hammers were pounding inside my brain. I didn't feel great but at least I could make an effort.

For one thing, the general-issue green hospital gown had to go. I'd had it on for three days now and I was fed up with it. Annette had brought me a T-shirt and shorts I'd spotted in the hotel the day we had arrived in Rio.

'What a rip-off,' I'd said when I noticed the price.

'They're lovely, though,' she'd replied.

We knew one of us would end up buying them and I had asked her to get them for me to cheer me up. At the time they had seemed a good souvenir of this trip; a white top with Rio in black letters across the chest and black shorts with Rio in white letters on one leg. They'd look great against a tan, though it seemed pretty unlikely that I'd get one of those now.

It was hard work being cheerful when I couldn't even dry my own hair. My hands were still numb and limp and that affected nearly everything I did. I had muddled my way through having a shower, although it had been hard turning the taps on and off. I couldn't tell whether the water was boiling hot or icy cold, either.

I was trying to put on some mascara when a nurse came in; she gently took the mascara wand from me and applied it for me, smiling. I'd been sitting in front of a little mirror in my room for ages trying to work out how to control my hands enough to lift the mascara to my eyes. It was impossible. I caught sight of myself in the mirror. God, you look like shit, I thought.

What had taken me all that morning to do would have been just the rushed start of an ordinary day a few days ago – taking a shower and getting dressed. I could feel tears of frustration burning at the back of my eyes. I didn't know what was wrong with me and I couldn't seem to do anything for myself. Where had the old me gone? It was as if the nurse understood even though we couldn't speak to each other. She stroked my face and left my room. I clambered up on to the bed. I turned to face the wall as I lay down, feeling scared and sorry for myself.

All I wanted to do was sleep. I felt as if whatever was making my body limp was doing the same to my mind. It frightened me that already I automatically used my hands to lift my feet and legs on to the bed or into place when I sat down. It was a change that seemed to have happened so quickly.

I'd left Craig a couple of days ago as an active, some might say hyperactive, young woman. Now I was like a little old lady, leaning heavily on whoever or whatever was close to hand and barely leaving my room except for the trek across the corridor to the bathroom.

What would he think when he saw me? Would he take one look and go away again? No, not Craig. He wasn't that type. He'd always been wonderful if I'd had a cold or flu and there was no reason to think he'd be any different now. I just longed to have his arms around me, then I'd know that nothing could harm me. But it was such a long way for him to come and he hated flying. I turned over in bed, the mattress springs and metal frame creaking. I couldn't believe my eyes.

'How long have you been there?' I asked. Craig smiled, his arms folded as he leaned against the doorpost. As he came walking towards me I could feel the relief flooding through me. *I wouldn't be alone any more.* I tried to smile back at him but instead I burst into tears and this time I thought the crying would never stop.

2. Diagnosis

As Craig walked across my room I could see that he was taking in every detail. We'd always said we could tell if something was wrong by looking into each other's eyes. Craig looked tired and drained and worried. This was going to be difficult. He's a buttoned-up sort of person; at times like this a peculiar quietness would grip him and I'd be left wondering if he cared. Of course he cared, he'd just flown thousands of miles through the night to be with me. Now it was my job to reassure him. So why was I sitting here crying? He sat on the edge of my bed, almost shy in this strange hospital room.

'My poor little Cazzy Mac,' he said, very quietly, as he put his arms around me. I suddenly felt safe, no harm would come to me. We sat for ages until the pain in my back was so intense I had to move.

'Don't worry, Craig, I'll be out of here soon,' I said, sniffing into his handkerchief. I wondered vaguely why his clothes were wet.

'I've brought your posh pyjamas, Caz,' he said to me, 'the blue silk ones with the lacy bits you like.'

'Thanks, honey. And where are the flowers and chocolates? A bunch of grapes? I'm a sick woman you know!'

'I'll go in search of everything your heart desires,' he said, 'and a packet of biscuits. I'm starving. But first, I must get these wet clothes off.'

Only Craig could have found a taxi driver who insisted on having all the windows open in the middle of a downpour. As the cab splashed through the streets from the airport poor Craig was soaked every time it drove through a puddle.

'There's no one anywhere, Caz,' he said. 'Is this a monsoon or something? The beach is empty, it's like a ghost town. You're not missing much in here.'

He began to tell me about his flight. I sat planning the best way to show him what my condition was really like. I looked quite good propped up in bed, my hair washed, my make-up in place. This time yesterday I'd looked such a wreck, if only he knew, I thought. Oh well, I'd better get it over with.

'I'll change in to those pyjamas,' I said, and lifted my legs across to the edge of the bed. They were a dead weight. I sat gathering my strength for the next stage of standing up.

'Please don't be shocked, Craig, it's just the numbness.' He looked away, busy finding a bag to put his wet clothes in.

'We'll get through this, Cazzy, don't you worry about that,' he said, looking up at the window as the rain suddenly started to beat down, spraying the windowsill. I'd left the window open a notch when the air conditioning had spluttered to a halt in the night. 'Doesn't it ever bloody stop raining in this place?' he shouted. 'Welcome to Rio!'

Poor Craig, he's more upset than I realized, I thought. This is going to be tricky. Then he smiled at me and came up with the perfect escape.

'I'll just run to the shop I passed on the way in and get some cigarettes while you're changing,' he said, leaving the room.

What I needed to do, I realized, was to make everything seem completely normal. What would Craig and I usually do when we met up again after one of my long-haul trips? Well, it hardly needs to be said. Under any other circumstances we'd have been in bed within minutes of seeing each other. We'd always had a good sex life.

'It's because we hardly ever see each other,' Craig had told friends of ours once when we'd been talking about keeping a relationship alive. 'Carole or I are always either just about to go somewhere or we've just come back from somewhere. And in-between we miss each other.'

His one dread was an ordinary girlfriend, someone at home with supper on the table every night. That would never do for Craig. But this time, this reunion really scared me. If I was numb from the shoulders down, would I be able to make love properly? It seemed unlikely, but I hadn't liked to ask Dr Fritz. It had been a bit, well, irrelevant, before Craig had arrived. Now it felt like the only thing that really mattered.

As I was struggling into my lovely silk pyjamas a nurse knocked on the door and pointed down the corridor. She helped me across the room. I steadied myself on the door frame and saw that a bigger room a few doors down was now empty. We were just packing my few odds and ends when Craig came back, loaded up with bottles of mineral water and the biggest packet of biscuits he could find. He'd already eaten half of them.

He took over and I went and lay on my new bed – still a single iron one, but the room itself was huge and it had two big improvements: there was an enormous fridge and the air conditioning worked. When the nurse had gone I realized it was time to face up to facts. I locked the door of my new room and Craig and I made love.

'I do love you, you know,' I said quietly. I felt so relieved; everything had been fine. As we lay on our sides wrapped around each other – clinging, really, to stop falling off the narrow bed – I smiled to myself. It hadn't been perfect, after all I had no feeling at all from the shoulders down. And anyway, neither of us was at our best. But at least things were in working order. God, how unromantic that sounds! Thank goodness Craig doesn't know what I'm thinking. It worried me that I hadn't felt I could discuss all of this with Craig, but he had only just arrived. I could already hear him breathing more and more softly as he fell asleep. He must be exhausted!

Suddenly, my legs started to shake, as though they didn't belong to me. Oh God, now what's happening? But it stopped as quickly as it had begun. I was glad Craig was asleep, I didn't want him panicking just yet.

When we woke up, just in time for dinner, my left side felt so weak that Craig had to cut up my food for me. We made a joke of it but I felt embarrassed. What must he think of me? This was all happening so quickly. But this wasn't the time for discussion; we were both tired so we settled into my little bed and were asleep within minutes.

The next thing I knew a nurse was creeping quietly into the room. It was morning; we'd slept for hours and hours. I tried to move but my arms were wrapped around Craig, who was still fast asleep. The nurse put one finger to her lips.

'Shh,' she said, and very gently lifted one of my arms, smiling at me. She quickly took a blood sample and wrapped my arm back around Craig, still smiling. As she tip-toed away she put her hands together as if in prayer then brought them up to the side of her face, leaning her head over on them. 'Sleep,' she said, 'sleep now.'

When Craig eventually woke up we embarked on a routine. There were tests, tests and more tests. Craig would break the monotony with splashes through the puddles to the grocer's shop.

As soon as he left the room I'd drag myself over to wherever he'd left his cigarettes, take one out and smoke it desperately, in deep drags, sitting up on top of the fridge and hanging out of the window like a naughty teenager! Hospital rules said no smoking, but what are a few rules when you're ill?

We were soon cracking up in that room and after three days Dr Fritz said we could move back to the hotel – on a few conditions. I wasn't to have hot baths, I mustn't go from extremes of temperature and I couldn't sit out in the sun.

'What sun?' I teased him, pointing out of the window to the lashing rain. At least they were all rules I could break and he would never know.

The journey over to the Rio Sheraton couldn't have been more different from the one I'd made, what, just a week ago? This time Copacabana Beach was empty, the sky grey and angry. The statue of Christ had disappeared, shrouded in mist. And I had needed help to get into the hospital car.

'Honestly, Craig. When I arrived last week this beach was packed. Where's the sunshine? It was scorching hot.' And I'd been able to jump on and off the crew bus, I thought.

'Perhaps the rain will clear and I'll get onto the beach after all, Caz.'

It was as though something earth-shattering had happened in the space of seven days. I shook my head. Don't be ridiculous, I told myself, all that's happened is that the weather has changed. You're becoming self-obsessed.

But that was hardly surprising. As the hall porter met us at the front entrance I realized that the wheelchair he was holding by its handles was for me. He gently helped me out of the car, holding my arm until I could sit down in the chair, then Craig wheeled me up the ramp to the front entrance.

I sat in the hotel lobby, the rain beating down on the glass roof, and realized I wasn't me any more. *I was me in a wheelchair.*

I was no longer the stewardess who strode through the door in her uniform, impatient to change into her shorts and order a gin and tonic. She wouldn't have noticed whether there was a wheelchair ramp or not. Why should she? I envied the me of a week ago.

A man in a terrible safari jacket, who had obviously packed for sunshine and not for rain, came walking towards the door. As Craig set off for the reception desk – pushing me in front of him – he ran over the poor man's toe. It was me who was treated to the angry look.

Don't blame me, it's Craig's fault, he's the driver, I felt like saying. It began to dawn on me how much control I had lost. He'd been here only a few days but I was becoming dependent on Craig.

Against all the odds we managed to have some fun once we were settled back at the Sheraton. Armed with an umbrella and the wheelchair we did wheelies along the abandoned sea front. I quite enjoyed being pushed everywhere. How lazy can a girl get?

On my first day back in the lap of luxury the neurologist lined up a real treat for me. I'm sure it was just to remind me that I might be out of hospital, but I wasn't out of the woods. If I'd known what was in store I might not have made the journey over to his clinic but by the time we arrived there it was too late to back out.

He glued electrodes into my hair and sent little currents of electricity whizzing through them. Poor Craig went quite pale when he realized what was going to happen.

'Do it to him!' I shouted out, laughing to cover up my nerves. Then the pain hit me. I want this game to end now, I thought. And as I looked up I noticed the nurse shaking her head. I was registering no reflex reaction at all. Things seemed to be looking worse rather than better. But still nobody could tell me what was wrong.

That night I woke up suddenly in a panic; I couldn't feel where my left arm was. I ripped back the duvet, sweating and breathing heavily. Oh God, it's not a nightmare, it's actually happening! I managed to sit upright, my feet hanging over the edge of the bed, and could see in the light from a crack in the curtain that yes, both my arms were still there! This was like going mad.

I realized that Craig hadn't woken up with me. He was fast asleep, even though the duvet was on the floor and I was sitting up panting in fear. Nobody sleeps that soundly, do they? Suddenly the penny dropped.

I dragged myself around the bed to his bedside drawer, very quietly opened it and rummaged around inside. A few handkerchiefs, a cigarette lighter, not what I was looking for. I slowly made my way into the bathroom, closed the door and turned on the light. As I rifled through his soap bag I found them – a bottle of sleeping pills, herbal ones. He must have bought them back home.

I realized for the first time how worried he was. How like us that we hadn't talked about it. He must have been worried sick, sitting back at my flat in Streatham, not knowing what was happening to me thousands of miles away. But he'd never said a word.

We had gone to a cabin crew party earlier that evening, and I'd seen the looks on the crew's faces as I'd scrambled out of my wheelchair and headed for a sofa.

'Poor Carole, what can I do to help her, I mustn't show how I feel,' seemed to flash through their minds. It actually came out as: 'So, Carole, what do the doctors say? Any nearer naming the mystery bug yet?'

Imagine what Craig must have been going through, waiting at home for a flight, not knowing what to expect when he arrived here, suddenly having a girlfriend who needs to have her dinner cut up. I sat on the edge of the bath and thought hard. There was only one thing to do, we would have to talk about this.

The next morning, down in the breakfast room, I fiddled with my red napkin and stared hard at the chequered pattern on the table-cloth.

'Craig, I found your sleeping tablets last night.' No answer. This was going to be harder than I'd thought.

'I was just wondering how long you've been taking them.'

'Oh, they're only herb things, not strong or anything,' he said, trying to avoid the issue.

'Yes, but why do you need them? You've never taken them before have you?'

'Look, Carole, what's the problem?' he said, suddenly irritated.

'My problem, Craig, is that I woke up in the middle of the night in a complete panic and an earthquake wouldn't have disturbed you.' Oh God, that sounded too selfish, too needy. I looked up.

'I'm sorry, Craig, I know you're worried about me, but could you come off the sleeping pills in case I need you? It's a lot to ask, but it would be a real help.'

'OK, Caz,' he said, as casually as if I'd asked him to pick up a newspaper on his way home.

This was all very Craig; I knew he'd do what I'd asked, but why did it always have to be so damn difficult to discuss anything important?

A few days later I was given permission to fly home. It was good to be back on board an aircraft. For me an airline cabin is a home from home, I feel safe when I'm flying. Business class was almost empty, which pleased me. I didn't want passengers to see me having my food cut up for me. It hadn't worried me in the hotel restaurant, but this seemed more real somehow. As we taxied down the runway, Craig buried his nose deep into a two-day-old *Daily Telegraph*, pretending it wasn't happening.

'Carole,' he whispered, 'what's that noise, is it normal?'

'It's the undercarriage, don't worry,' I told him in what had become our ritual when we flew together. Perhaps it's because I love flying so much, but I can't believe he's such a nervous flier.

'Caz, what's that noise?' he asked again, a few seconds later. This went on and on until just before take-off.

'What's that noise?' he asked one last time.

'It means we're going to crash, Craig,' I answered him, laughing. Then I saw the look on his face. 'I'm only joking, we're OK,' I said.

'Honestly, Craig, fancy being scared of flying and going out with a stewardess!'

For the first time in several weeks, I was the stronger one and I enjoyed having that feeling back.

'Tell you what, Craig, we'll come back to Rio when I'm better and get some serious sunbathing done.'

I smiled at him. I was glad he'd come out to Rio; just by being there and giving support he had helped more than he will ever know. There was no reply from him now, though; the plane was just lifting up in to the sky and it would be some minutes before he would be capable of talking.

Back home, I was no longer an emergency and had to wait my turn for an appointment with a neurologist. I hadn't expected that; somehow I thought I'd be a priority as nobody had yet diagnosed what was wrong.

In the meantime the shock of leaving hotel life behind – with an army of staff cooking my meals, cleaning my room and doing the washing up – had forced me to face up to just how ill I was. At first I had Craig there to check the temperature of my bath. I couldn't tell whether it was boiling hot or ice cold. He could drive me around, too, so I wasn't entirely housebound. My Jeep was still at Heathrow airport, parked where I'd left it on the way out to Rio.

My dad came up from Devon to see me. What father wouldn't be concerned when his 23-year-old daughter has to ask him to tie up her shoelaces? I told him about all the tests I'd had in Rio but every time I told my story now I worried what it sounded like. I tried going for a walk with him on Wimbledon Common – my first fresh air, really, for weeks. But I needed to get back home. I felt uncomfortable outdoors in an open space. Perhaps I was trying to pretend that things were better than they really were.

I was beginning to worry that everyone must be thinking I was a hypochondriac. They were hard weeks, trying not to worry everyone unnecessarily, and inside feeling more worried than I'd ever been in my life. My world shrank, too. If I wanted to go anywhere, I would need to use a wheelchair, so I didn't bother to go anywhere. I could walk around my flat, but I kept banging into things and when I stood up I had the weirdest sensation that I was going to fall over. It was all so new and unpredictable.

' We both knew that Craig would soon be going away. I didn't want to make a big deal of it. Anyway, doctors are trained to make us better so I never doubted for a second that I would soon be diagnosed and cured. I believed that anything which struck as quickly as this had must be a virus and that it would disappear just as suddenly. Even so, in the week before he went I cried every day.

There was no question that I would ask him not to go, and there was equally no way that he'd have chosen to stay with me. It's fair to say Craig lives for golf and his new post at a new course near Helsinki was perfect for him. The pay was good and once he was out there he'd be in his element.

He booked a cab and when the buzzer rang for him, I stood in the kitchen, crying. We had always hated saying goodbye, so I never even walked to the front door to see him go. He opened the front door, then came back in and held me tight.

'I hate it when you have to go,' I said to him, and he left suddenly, without saying a word.

The front door slammed shut and there was silence in the flat. Then I noticed an envelope propped up on the work top in the kitchen. Inside was a card: 'I love you so much, I miss you,' he'd written. He was good at things like that, but this was too much for me.

'What did he have to do that for?' I shouted out. I held out my hand to steady myself against the doorframe, put my other hand on the back of a chair and sat down. I was scared and lonely. I didn't know when I would next see Craig and I didn't understand why this virus couldn't be given a name and cured. I felt so sorry for myself. A month ago I'd been fine. Now I didn't know what was happening to me. I laid my head on my arms and cried and cried, the sound echoing round the empty flat.

I was staring at Dr Fritz's notes on me, the results of all the many tests he'd done. 'Good luck, Carole, and take care,' he'd said as he had handed them over on my last appointment with him in Rio. Now here they were, stacked up on Dr Pauline Monro's desk at Bolingbroke Hospital in Wandsworth.

'Tell me what happened in Rio, Carole,' she said, brushing her fingers through her white hair as I sat down opposite her.

'Well, there are all the tests they did, haven't you read my notes?' I asked, waving towards the folders.

'Yes, I have, but I want to hear your version,' she said, kindly. So I told her my story, mentioning a new symptom that had started a few days ago, a buzzing that started at the top of my spine and sort of fizzed all the way down my back.

'Does it happen when you bend your head forward?' she asked.

'I don't know,' I replied.

'Well, try it, would you please,' she said. I eased my head forward and the most horrific sensation flooded down my spine. I was amazed. How on earth did she know that would happen?

'So what do you think is wrong with me?' I asked her.

'There's a possibility it could be inflammation of the nervous system,' she replied, looking me straight in the eye. That doesn't sound too bad, I thought, a few antibiotics and I'll get back to normal.

'Now, Carole, I want you to get booked in for an MRI scan,' she said.

'A what?' Not more tests! 'I don't think there's any inch of me that hasn't been put to the test,' I said, and for the first time since I'd met her, Dr Monro smiled.

I went home and waited. In Rio I'd had to rely on Dr Fritz to tell me everything, but here on home ground I could do my own homework. The MRI, or Magnetic Resonance Imaging, scanner was brand new – a huge contraption, linked to a computer, that would take pictures of my brain and spinal cord. I had no idea why they wanted to do that, but if it got me nearer to a diagnosis I'd do anything.

I didn't feel so brave when I got to the Churchill Clinic in south London and actually saw the thing. It looked like a huge white wall with a large hole in it, almost like a modern work of art. I had to be strapped into a bed and the bed then slid into that hole, like a CD slipping into a giant CD player.

My friend Liz had come with me to this clinic; in fact, she'd driven me everywhere since Craig had left. She's a head-turning blonde and the most practical person you could meet. Her toddler Kurt usually came with us, but today we'd left him at home with his dad so she was free to mother me! It was just as well.

'I don't like the look of this, Liz,' I said. I could feel my heart begin to race. As the padding went around my head and a bar snapped into place across my waist it was like getting on to a rollercoaster lying down. A nurse put a panic button into my hand.

'If you feel scared, Carole, just press this and we'll have you out of there in seconds,' she said, smiling.

Panic set in on the first attempt, and on the second. The nurse gave me an injection of Valium. By now I didn't have any padding; she'd taken it all off after the first try. I was under strict instructions to keep my head absolutely still, a bit like smiling for the camera. Liz walked round to the other side of the wall, sat by my head and kept chattering about nothing. But I was away, lying on a beach beneath a huge golden sun, and didn't listen to her at all.

The Valium kept me inside the scanner for the full 25 minutes as the machinery clanged and clattered and took its pictures. But even under sedation I could feel the terror of being trapped. I kept repeating: 'Get these bars off me, I've got to get out!'

At last it was over and poor Liz, at a loss to know what to do to help, drove me home. It wasn't until that evening, at dinner with friends and in the middle of a conversation about house prices of all things, that I suddenly burst into tears. It was the only time I ever allowed myself to be given Valium to get through anything. Why bother with a drug that just delays the inevitable?

I felt shaky and low after the scan. I'd been home from Rio for two months by now and it was time for some pampering. All I really wanted to do was fly out to Finland to be with Craig, but as the hospital asked me to stay in the country I settled for a trip to see my dad down in Tiverton. It was May, a lovely month to be in Devon.

He had lived there for a couple of years since splitting up with my mum, and had a beautiful home, very peaceful. I took a train from Paddington station in west London, determined that I didn't need help – and definite that I didn't need a wheelchair. It sounds an easy trip, but by the time I got off the train in Bristol I was shaking with exhaustion.

The effort of carrying my suitcase sent pain flooding out from my spine, down my arms and along my shoulders. People were rushing past me, racing for their trains. As I reached the front of the station, with its honey-coloured walls and cloistered entrance, Dad's car swung in to view. I'd been grown-up for long enough. I dropped my suitcase, sat down on it, and with my head in my hands burst into tears. Getting here had been like climbing Everest.

'Sweetheart,' I heard him cry across the taxi rank in front of me, 'what's wrong?' We were putting on our seat belts when he turned to me and said: 'Where does it hurt, poppet?'

'Oh, Dad, it's my back, and my arms hurt now as well.'

'Let's get home and you can have a good rest,' he said and as we drove through the Devon countryside I knew I'd made the right decision to come. As my stay went on and he bustled around in the kitchen and fussed after me, I learnt a simple truth: when you're ill you need care. You can't do it all alone. I lay on the sofa looking out across his immaculate garden to the fields in the distance and realized that without this illness, whatever it was, I would never have given him the chance to spoil me like this.

I went home feeling better than I'd been for ages. Dr Monro had given me a date for my diagnosis at last. I was desperate to know what was wrong with me. Lying in bed alone at night I had started to wonder whether the symptoms were in my head. Surely one of the hundreds of tests I'd had would have shown them what it was by now?

I knew, in my heart, there *would* be a name for whatever it was I had. For one thing, the numbness was real. And I was missing my independence too much to be making this up. I'd have given anything to have my Jeep back and be able to go where I liked, on my own. I was hardly the type to put my job in danger, either. I loved my work and although British Airways was being very supportive I knew that couldn't last for ever. Why should it? I needed to put a name to whatever it was that was happening to me.

A few days before I was due to see Dr Monro, I had a sure sign that I was on the mend. I was sitting in the bath – I used a thermometer now to check that the water wasn't too hot – and as I washed myself I realized I could feel my right hip. I prodded and poked and yes, normal sensation had come back. I clambered out of the bath, and still dripping wet and in my bath robe, phoned Craig.

'Good news, honey,' I said, ' the numbness is beginning to go away, things are looking up.'

'That's great, Caz,' he said, 'so when will you be able to come out here?'

'When I know the test results,' I said. 'I'll phone as soon as Dr Monro tells me what's wrong. I can't wait to see you.'

Dr Monro was at the Atkinson Morley Hospital in Wimbledon on the day of our appointment. It's a friendly, old-fashioned little cottage hospital, and I thought it suited the doctor perfectly. I was relieved when I woke up that at last my diagnosis had come through. It was a lovely day, 6 June 1991, with a bright blue sky. A good omen, I thought, none of that dreadful greyness I'd had in Rio in those first dark days.

I had decided to go to the hospital by taxi, so my friend Liz said she'd wait at my flat for me to hear the news when I returned. As I drew up at the front entrance I suddenly felt that I hadn't a care in the world. I knew I was getting better very slowly and assumed the doctor was going to tell me that I was over the worst. My left side was still weak but my walking was improving every day and I felt stronger. I went through the entrance and stood chatting to the receptionist, all the time thinking how desperate I was to hear this diagnosis.

So it came as a real surprise when I went into Dr Monro's tiny consulting room and she asked me to undress and go through the door to her examination room.

'There are just a few more tests, Carole, if you'll bear with me.'

I was stunned. She hasn't been able to find out what it is, I thought. After all this time, she still doesn't know. My eyes felt hot with tears. I was obviously more keyed-up than I'd realized. The truth is, I felt I would go mad if I had to leave the hospital without a name for whatever was wrong with me.

The look on Dr Monro's face was completely blank. She wasn't giving anything away as she tested my eyes, again, and my reflexes, again. She even made me walk across the floor, just like the neurologist that first afternoon in my hotel room in Rio three months before. I felt I'd been doing the same old tests again ever since.

'Thank you, Carole, if you'd put your clothes back on now? Then I'd like a word with you.'

I'd worn nothing but track suits for weeks. They have no buttons and they're easy to put on and take off. So I was soon walking through to join Dr Monro where she was sitting at her desk, her head bent over my files. As I sat down she tidied them in to a neat pile then looked up, almost shyly.

'We've had the results from your scan, Carole,' she said.

Thank goodness. Now we're getting somewhere, I thought.

'All my tests have led me to believe that you do have inflammation of the nervous system.' For a split second, I felt real frustration.

'Well, if that's all, what can you do to make me better? How do I get rid of it?' I asked. Inflammation, infection, antibiotics? It should be easy, I thought.

'Look, Dr Monro, I've waited long enough. It's been three months. I really need to know exactly what is wrong with me.'

It sounded simple but I was disturbed by the tone in her voice. Was it my imagination, I thought, or had it suddenly gone quieter? I felt as though I couldn't breathe. Everything seemed to be winding down in to slow motion.

She must have been dreading this moment, but Dr Monro looked me straight in the eyes and explained: 'I'm afraid, Carole, that inflammation of the nervous system is multiple sclerosis.'

3. Time to Think

What a relief, I thought, as Dr Monro and I sat looking at each other. At last, this thing has a name and I can start dealing with it. I'll get leaflets, read books, find out everything I can, get to grips with all of this ...

'Do you know what multiple sclerosis is, Carole?' Dr Monro asked, her voice cutting through my thoughts.

'Wheelchair,' I replied and then cleared my throat. The sound of my own voice seemed to belong to someone else. I can't have multiple sclerosis because I can't be seriously ill, I thought.

'Carole, I would like our counsellor to talk to you,' said Dr Monro. 'She can answer all your questions and tell you everything you need to know.'

'I don't want to see a counsellor, thanks. I want to be on my own and I want to have a cup of coffee and a cigarette.' I felt so calm you'd have thought we were discussing the weather.

I was shown to the canteen by the receptionist I'd been chatting to, what, 15 minutes ago? It seemed like a previous life.

'Come back up in your own time, Carole, and the counsellor will be there if you need her,' she told me, then left.

I poured myself a coffee, something I couldn't have done a few weeks before. Both of my hands had been numb then, hadn't they? Will I be that useless all the time eventually? I wondered. I went over to an orange-topped table, as far away from a couple chatting quietly by the coffee machine as I could go. I turned my back on them and sat down, lit a cigarette and realized that my hands were completely steady. Perhaps I'm in shock, I thought, looking out of the window at a scrap of garden more weeds than lawn.

I don't know how long I stayed there, running it over and over in my head. I couldn't believe the diagnosis. It was literally unbelievable. I had just turned 24, doing everything I wanted to do, life was good. So why me? Why now? Why multiple sclerosis? No, it must be wrong. I suddenly needed to go home. I didn't want to talk to anyone, but I did want to read something about this condition. I stubbed out my cigarette and made my way back to the reception area. Waiting there was a young pregnant woman who stood up as I approached and smiled across at me.

'Carole?' she inquired. When I nodded, she waved towards a room I had just walked past. 'Let's go in there,' she said.

We settled into low plastic-covered armchairs – in fact, too low for the counsellor who managed to smile at me as she flopped down heavily.

'My name is Ashley Green, Carole. Now is there anything you want to ask me about what the doctor has told you this morning?' she said.

'No, but I want some leaflets,' I answered. There was a slight pause as we looked at each other.

'Will I be able to have children?'

'Yes, but it's better to do it earlier rather than later.' She instinctively put a protective hand across her own belly. 'The stress of giving birth can trigger a relapse. Everyone's different, though. You might be fine.'

'Will I lose my job?' I asked, wondering where such clear-headed thinking was coming from.

'I don't know.' She gave me a sympathetic glance as she passed over a handful of pamphlets. I looked down at them.

'Can I have sex?' I asked her, and looked up. This time we both smiled.

'Yes, but try to do it when you're most awake, perhaps in the afternoon for example.'

We both laughed but quickly fell silent again. 'Carole, are you sure you're OK?' she asked.

'I'm fine,' I said. 'I just want to go home.'

Sitting in the taxi my mind started to race. I realized that at some time during the day I would have to tell everyone. They all knew that this was my diagnosis day; I'd been so keyed-up that I had hardly talked about anything else recently. My mum was my first concern. It was going to be hard for her. She loved living in Australia, but she'd want to be with me, to help me. Any mother would feel the same with a child who'd just been given such news. Then there was Craig in Finland, and my dad was away on a business trip to Scotland. And I'd have to tell British Airways. Or would I? Perhaps I should keep quiet. No, I didn't have a choice. But would I lose my job if I were honest with them? And my sister, Hazel, nannying in Switzerland. Where's her phone number? It's in my Filofax somewhere. God, everything was so complicated suddenly. How the hell was I going to tell everyone?

Liz was sitting in the flat with little Kurt playing on the floor in the living-room as I walked in. She jumped up.

'So, what did she say, Carole?' she asked. 'What did the doctor say?'

I started to grin, I think with nerves. 'You're not going to believe this,' I began, but I couldn't say any more. I littered the leaflets across the floor for her to see and sank into the sofa sobbing. Just at that moment my neighbour rang and Liz calmly asked her to call back later. Then, without saying a word, she collected up the leaflets and started to look at them.

The flat was silent – even Kurt sensed that this was no time to make a noise. He just sat on the floor staring first at me then at his mum. I didn't want to talk and I couldn't really think of anything to say. After a while all I wanted was to be alone. I felt as though I had so much to do. While I was sitting there I decided I had to go to Finland immediately.

'I don't want to tell Craig over the phone,' I said out loud, but inside I was thinking: 'What will he do? What will he think?'

'Well, it might do you good to go out to see him, Carole,' Liz said gently. She didn't know how to react, what to say or what to do.

'Thanks for being here,' I said, 'but do you mind if I have some time on my own now? I've so much to do!' She looked slightly relieved and within seconds she had packed away Kurt's toys and was standing at the front door.

'Look, anything you want, just call me,' said Liz, ever practical as she kissed me on the cheek. I stood waving at Kurt while he was being strapped into his car seat then shut the front door. Silence. Right, I thought, first things first. I must phone BA.

'My God, Carole, I'm so sorry,' said my manager David Barton as soon as I told him.

'Am I going to lose my job?' I asked, trying to remain calm.

'You'll have to see the doctors,' he said, 'but don't worry.'

'I have to go to Finland tomorrow, David,' I said. 'I'm on standby for a seat at the moment but it's almost full. I must be on that flight.'

'We'll get you on it, even if you're sitting on the flight deck. Look, Carole, take two weeks to talk things through with Craig and don't even think about work. Just turn up tomorrow morning and I'll make sure the crew know why you're making the trip. You'll be on board, no matter what.'

I was in automatic mode by now. I rang to make an appointment with BA's chief of medical services. She would be the person who decided whether or not I could continue flying. Every time I put down the phone it rang as my friends and family called to hear what had happened.

'I have MS,' I kept saying, and each time it seemed as though I was talking about someone else. Then my mum rang.

'Hello darling, how did you get on with your doctor today?' she asked. She sounded tired and I glanced at my watch. I realized she had stayed up till the early hours of the morning in Perth to make the call.

'They think I have multiple sclerosis, Mum,' I said. There was a silence as the time delay gave us both a few seconds to keep our voices under control. I was determined that there would be no tears, no weeping on the phone. It just wasn't fair on her as she was so far away.

'Oh Carole, I wish I could be there with you,' she said. 'I love you so much. I should be with you. You need somebody to look after you.'

'Don't worry, Mum, I'm going to Finland tomorrow to be with Craig.'

'Good, I'm really glad. I don't like to think of you on your own. I hate feeling that I'm not doing anything for you.' She rang off. The truth was that her life was in Australia with her husband Ivan and there was nothing she could do for me.

I was very matter-of-fact with my dad and my voice must have sounded so calm that it worried him.

'Do you realize how serious this is?' he asked. I could hear the low buzz of men's voices in the background. He must have called during a break in his conference.

'Of course I do, Dad.' I felt a little put out. Later in the day he rang back.

'I'm worried that you haven't quite taken it all in, poppet,' he said. He sounded shocked and I thought how hard it must be for him, trying to make it through a working day with this on his mind. But Dad wasn't the only one who rang back. Several friends did, too, just to make sure they'd heard me right the first time.

Then Craig rang. I was determined not to break my news to him over the phone.

'I've sorted out a flight for tomorrow morning, Craig,' was all I said. 'I'll tell you about it when I see you.'

'No. Tell me now, honey,' he replied. I knew he had no one with him in Finland. I wanted him to read all of my leaflets and to be with him so that we could get used to this together.

'In two words, Caz. Tell me what the doctor said.'

'Multiple sclerosis,' I said. There was a pause.

'You must be joking.'

We both fell silent. This was not what I had wanted.

'No, I'm not joking, Craig. I'll see you tomorrow. We can talk about it then. Don't worry, I'll explain everything when I see you.'

I needed to get some order into my life, do the practical things, keep a cool head. I'd have time to deal with the emotional stuff in Finland. Now I was concerned about Craig and worried about everyone I had spoken to on the phone. So I switched off. What did

I need to do? Pack and get out to Finland. Everything else could wait.

At last the phone stopped ringing and I had time to myself. I ran a bath and thought about Craig. I'd wanted to tell him face to face but he'd messed up my plans. What was he doing right now? I was so excited about seeing him. He'd been away for six weeks. I had never been to his new golf course so I couldn't even imagine where he was sitting or walking or what his house was like. He'd be great at the practical side of things with me. Look how good he was with the wheelchair out in Rio. But emotionally, how would he cope with the thought of me permanently in a wheelchair?

I clambered out of the bath. It was strange. I'd learned I was seriously ill just as the feeling was coming back to most of my body and my co-ordination was improving. In my bath robe, with a cup of coffee and a cigarette, I sat at my dining table and shuffled the leaflets the counsellor had given me. I'd better know what this is all about before I saw Craig or I wouldn't be able to answer his questions. I realized that I didn't know anybody with MS, so it was these leaflets or nothing. I picked up a bright pink booklet and opened the first page.

Diagnosed with MS? When you are first told that you have MS you are likely to feel shocked and bewildered. That was true enough. I think I had been in shock for most of the day. It had never crossed my mind that I'd be diagnosed with a serious illness. The sense of relief I'd felt at first had worn off already. I turned back to the leaflet.

The most common age of diagnosis is late twenties to mid-thirties. Well, that wasn't fair. I was only 23 in Rio. Why had it got me so young?

MS is a chronic condition of the central nervous system. The central nervous system is the brain and spinal cord. Oh my God. A chronic condition. Please not this, not multiple sclerosis, I kept thinking.

The symptoms experienced with MS are caused by demyelination, or scarring, in the central nervous system. It is not yet known what actually triggers off the process of scarring. So, nobody knows why I've got MS? What about the symptoms? I wanted to see how they were described.

Symptoms of MS. There is no set pattern to MS and some people will experience symptoms which others will not. However, some symptoms are common for many people:

- *Blurring of vision, double vision.* No, I'd never had that.
- *Weakness or clumsiness of a limb.* I'd had that since Rio, except all of my limbs had felt weak and floppy, and sort of heavy. Like I was dragging my feet around.
- *Tingling or numbness in arms or legs.* Yup, I had that.
- *Giddiness or lack of balance.* Yes.
- *Fatigue which is out of proportion to what you have done, or unpredictable fatigue.* I couldn't remember not feeling tired, really.
- *The need to pass water frequently and/or urgently.* Oh God,that one hasn't struck yet.

Reading this stuff was beginning to freak me out. I obviously needed to deal with it slowly and I'd done enough for one day. There was no need to keep going. I went to bed and fell asleep straight away, out cold. I was exhausted but at least I'd be with Craig tomorrow.

My manager was as good as his word. The crew on the flight to Helsinki all knew what had happened and why I needed to go to Finland so urgently. I didn't say anything about my illness to anyone.

'Carole, we thought you'd like some champagne,' one stewardess said to me, pouring a glass as soon as the plane was in the air. It was the first of several, and as I relaxed and went up to the flight deck for a chat with the pilots I suddenly felt happy. I was going to have Craig to myself for two weeks and with him there everything would be fine.

I had a suitcase half-filled with slushy books and this was going to be a fabulous holiday, a real escape. The crew must have thought I was mad, or that the manager had made a mistake, but as we landed I was grinning from ear to ear. There was that familiar rush of excitement when I was about to see Craig and not even multiple sclerosis could take that away from me.

Craig was in love with Finland. He'd described it to me as peaceful and tranquil and as I spotted him through the glass partition in the arrivals hall at Helsinki airport he looked more relaxed and happy than I'd seen him for months and months. I waved furiously and as I rushed towards the exit I bashed my trolley into a harrassed-looking woman with three children in tow.

'I'm so sorry,' I shouted back over my shoulder and then ran towards Craig and threw myself at him.

We kissed and hugged each other for so long that the passengers from my flight had all disappeared by the time Craig was pushing my trolley towards the exit to the car park.

'So it's MS then eh, Caz?' he asked as we walked side by side.

'So they say.' There was silence as we made our way to his car.

'You're going to love this place,' he said.

The road was so straight that I could see hundreds of yards ahead. The reflection of the pine trees on either side made odd shapes and patterns on the car's windscreen and even though the sky was blue and the sun was shining, the dark green forest made everything seem quiet and muffled.

'How far is it, Craig?' I asked, my usual question at the start of any journey.

'It's about an hour's drive,' he said. 'Hey Caz, you're looking great,' he added, smiling.

'You're looking good yourself, Craig. How's it been out here? You're having the time of your life, aren't you?'

'I can't wait to show you my house. You'll love it.'

Yesterday's diagnosis started to seem unreal and I realized it was my job to make it real for Craig. We needed this time alone to plan ahead and I had a lot of thinking to do. Out here it would be so simple to pretend that nothing had happened to me.

As we turned off the road and made our way up a newly-laid track I could see his house in the distance. He was living in the middle of nowhere. No wonder Craig was happy, this situation was tailor-made for him.

He had the ground floor of a house that had been built with the St

Laurence golf course. The course wound its way around the house. From every one of the windows draped with cream blinds you could see golfers making their way around the course, and beyond them just more forest. I went from window to window.

'Craig, it's perfect,' I said and I started to drag a huge rocking chair across the wooden floor of the main room. 'Now tell me where you work most of the time.'

He walked over to one of the windows and pointed at the golf range. 'That's where I give most of my lessons,' he said.

'Then that's the best view for me. Every time I look up while I'm reading, you'll be there.' I pushed the chair into place, unlocked my suitcase and put a pile of books on the window sill. 'I've arrived,' I said, and we went out for a stroll.

I knew we had to sit down and talk about MS. It didn't feel strained at all, even though there was one very important option I needed to put to Craig.

'How are you feeling about everything, Craig?' I asked that evening after we'd cooked up some pasta and sauce on the Aga. We were sitting at the scrubbed kitchen table and I went over to my bag and sorted out my leaflets.

'To be honest, Caz, I'm more worried about how you're feeling.'

'Look, Craig, why don't you read these and then ask me anything about them that you don't understand?'

I put the leaflets down on the table. Craig glanced over at them and nodded. I remembered some of what was in them. *MS is a chronic condition ... It is impossible to predict with certainty how MS is going to affect an individual in the future.* I thought I'd better say what had really been on my mind since I'd come out of Dr Monro's office yesterday morning.

'I don't know what my future holds any more, Craig. If you're going to leave, do it now. Don't wait,' I said, looking at him, then at the table.

'Why on earth would I want to go?' he replied.

'MS is unpredictable, Craig. Do you think you could cope with not knowing what's going to happen to me next?'

'Don't be so ridiculous, Caz, you know I love you. Don't worry. Everything is going to be fine.'

It was the answer I had expected. I had never doubted his love for one minute, but this was new territory for both of us. The rest of the evening was wonderful. The setting was perfect, and as the daylight extended into the night it gave me a rush of energy and I felt better than I had for weeks.

We always needed to spend a night together before we could relax properly in each other's company and by the time Craig went off for a lesson at nine o'clock the next morning I felt I really was on holiday. I snuggled down into the bed and went straight back to sleep. Here there was perfect peace. Hours later, when Craig came home for lunch, I was still sleeping. He went away again. When I finally woke up all I did was to make some coffee and curl up in the rocking chair to read.

The leaflets lay on the kitchen table, untouched.

After that first night, I had no energy for the first few days in Finland. It was as if the past months were catching up with me. There was no telephone in the house, the television was in Finnish, of course, although I did watch several old British movies with subtitles. I felt completely detached.

The next evening Craig wanted to show me around the golf course but after walking for three or four holes I felt shaky and exhausted. I thought he would read the leaflets when we went back to the house. I would have done had things been the other way around. I could deal with everyone else when I went home, but this was our time. It was important that we talked about this now so that we could face whatever was coming together.

But the leaflets stayed where I'd put them.

After three or four days, this was starting to make me angry. I felt he didn't care and I could feel resentment building up inside me. I'm having to deal with all this, why won't you? I kept thinking. Then I confronted him.

'Craig, please read those leaflets, I need you to help me with this,' I said, trying to keep my voice light and casual. 'I need your support.'

'OK, Caz, I'll do it tomorrow,' he replied.

I looked into his eyes and I thought I could see fear there. Perhaps he was scared to read about this illness that had turned my life upside down.

'I don't want to read about what might never happen to you,' he went on. 'I want us to deal with things when they happen, together, as a couple.'

'OK, Craig,' I said.

'You said yourself that it's going to be unpredictable, Caz. You might never have any more symptoms.'

His decision put pressure on me from that day on. If he didn't know what the symptoms of MS were, I would always have to describe them. I could feel frustration creeping in. Craig had chosen not to inform himself about my illness and I wondered whether there would always be a right time to tell him if I was experiencing a new symptom.

I could eat a meal without needing any help by now and my co-ordination was almost as good as new. The more I rested, the more I would try to do, and then my symptoms would return. It was like taking two steps forward and one step back all the time. One day we went for a walk on the golf course then went back to the house and made love. My legs went into spasm which lasted 10 minutes. We both laughed it off but it was a shock as I realized my limits.

'It's one or the other, Craig,' I said. 'If you want the sex, forget the walk. Both in one day is just too much!'

'That's fine by me, Caz.' We both laughed again.

Craig hates flying and I had never liked golf. One day when I was reading at my window, I looked up and saw Craig painstakingly teaching a teenage boy how to hold his club. It was time I learned to play. He gave me a club and some balls and I went off to a quiet corner to practise in private.

'Excuse me,' I heard a tiny voice from behind me after about 10 minutes. I turned around and a little boy, I would guess he was about six years old, was watching me. It appeared he was trying to tell me something in Finnish.

'Hello,' I said, looking to see if his mum or dad were nearby. Perhaps he needed help to find his way back to the clubhouse, 'do you speak English?'

'Yes, a little.'

'What's your name?'

'Christopher,' he replied. 'I think you hold your golf club badly.' His voice was so sweet and so serious that I almost burst out laughing.

'Would you show me?' I asked him, and as he demonstrated his swing, biting his lip in concentration, I realized that golf wasn't for me. I'm too impatient.

I had no choice but to rest on that holiday. I could see Craig all the time from the house, somewhere out on the course teaching a never-ending stream of pupils. We went into the nearest town, Lohja, a few times and we had dinner with some English friends. But we never confronted the subject of multiple sclerosis. I tried several times and Craig always changed the subject.

'Don't worry, Caz, everything will be fine.' He must have said it a dozen times. He didn't seem to understand that things weren't going to be fine this time. As the two weeks went on, I felt more and more alone. I was no longer the person Craig had met and fallen in love with. I had always been the caring one, looking after him, cooking his dinner and being totally independent. Now I needed help and he wasn't giving it to me.

The oddest thing was that I never cried about MS. I wanted Craig to put his arms around me so that I could cry. If he'd been stronger, I'd have done that but he made me feel that I mustn't fall apart in front of him. We never cried about it together so we could never move on and face this thing, this terrible illness, together. During my second week in Finland I cried every day at the thought of going home. Perhaps I was crying about Craig and me really. It's better to get all those feelings out into the open and out of the way but I felt that Craig had denied me the opportunity to do that.

One day I went to the clubhouse and rang my mum from the public phone beside the terraced bar. Golfers were sunning themselves over a glass of beer. I wanted her to know that I was well and having a good time.

'Hello, Mum, this is just a very quick call. Craig's fine and I'm feeling much better,' I said in my happiest voice. 'This is a beautiful place, Mum, you'd love Finland.'

'I'm so pleased you're OK, Carole,' she said.

A pattern was beginning to take shape; not crying, not admitting my fears, not talking to people honestly and properly.

I hated the drive to the airport when one of us was leaving. Craig always cracked appalling jokes, cheering me up because he knew I never wanted to leave him.

'Make the most of it, Caz, I'll be home before you know it,' he said as he turned the car out onto the main road. 'Then you can moan about me leaving my clothes all over the flat and not doing the washing-up!'

'Not this time, Craig, I'm not in the mood,' I said. I resented him being in Finland and I was angry about all my leaflets in his kitchen, knowing full well that he wasn't going to touch them.

It's strange, I thought, two weeks ago I'd been so happy to be here. We'd had each other to ourselves the whole time, with no interruptions from the usual endless stream of phone calls Craig hated so much from my friends. But I felt that we'd lost something. I didn't love him any less, but the holiday had made me aware of a problem that we had; as a couple we couldn't communicate with each other. I'd never noticed it before but I suppose we'd never faced a major problem before.

As we drove along yet another straight uncomplicated road my head was buzzing with worries. Craig had never once offered to give up his post in Finland, and I needed him to be with me. But I would never ask him to give this up; he was so happy and if he came home he'd be miserable. I didn't want to go home alone to face all the changes I was going through, though. I was broke, too. I had a mortgage and I hadn't been to work for more than three months. I was down to basic pay now and I feared even that would stop soon.

'I'm really worried about my job, Craig,' I said, almost as though I was breaking in on my own thoughts. 'What do you think BA is going to do when I go home?'

'Don't worry about it, Caz, it'll turn out fine, you'll see.'

'But what if it doesn't, Craig, what will I do then?'

'Look, Caz, they're not going to sack you are they?'

'I don't know.'

'Wait and see what their doctors say. You can't do anything till then, so there's no point worrying about it.'

He didn't have a clue! He was earning good money, loved Finland and had thoroughly enjoyed having me all to himself for two weeks.

By the time we reached Helsinki airport I was sobbing. I wanted to scream at Craig: 'Don't you understand, *I'm scared!*' Instead I clung on to him and didn't want to let go. How different all of this was, I thought. It was as though someone else was doing all these things, not me. I'd always been so independent. Now look at me!

'I'll see you soon, Caz,' Craig said as my flight was called. 'I'll be home in a few months. Don't worry. Things will turn out OK. I love you so much.'

Nothing had filtered through to him. Things would never turn out OK because I had multiple sclerosis. He would leave the airport, go back to his golf and it would be as if none of this had happened.

The flight was too long, really. Perhaps I'd had too much time to myself in Finland, thinking. Now I had another three-and-a-half hours alone with my thoughts. I started to cry again.

'Would you like a sweet, madam?' a stewardess asked me. She probably thought I was scared of flying. A sweet, for God's sake! It was going to take a lot more than that to make me feel better.

'No thanks,' I said, trying to find a tissue. 'I'll be fine in a minute.'

For the first time since I'd been diagnosed, I started to feel really anxious. What's going to happen next? Am I going to end up in a wheelchair? Which part of my body will be affected? And for how long? It was a nightmare being stuck with my thoughts on that journey.

I also had to face the fact that Craig had disappointed me. I didn't want a father figure, but nor did I want to be a mother figure. If I was going to fight this illness I needed an equal partner, and we weren't equals. He was refusing to educate himself about the biggest thing that had ever happened to either of us. I was coming home knowing that I was on my own in this fight.

We landed at Heathrow and I walked off the plane into a wall of heat. It was so humid I could hardly breathe. Helsinki had been heaven compared with this. I could feel my energy draining out of me. I had nowhere to hide now. The holiday was over and it was time to start looking reality in the face, however terrifying and uncertain it was.

As I walked into the airport terminal I knew my life was never going to be normal again. But if it wasn't going to be normal, what would it be like? I felt scared when I realized I had no idea.

4. Back to Work

Instead of being told I was about to die, I'd been told I had to start living with a disease that could suddenly get worse. Dr Monro hadn't sat me down to say: 'I'm sorry, Carole, but you have six months to live.' There was no pattern to what was coming. I didn't need to rush around doing the things I'd always wanted to do. Yet it wasn't as though I could go to see somebody and they'd tell me what my life was going to be like. I'd never met anyone with multiple sclerosis and even if I had I already realized that my MS would be unique. Even my doctor didn't have any answers. I was on my own.

I'd spent the months since Rio worrying about my diagnosis but all the time real life had been carrying on. For one thing, I was in debt. I hadn't worked for three months and the bills were piling up. I had been earning good money flying long-haul so I'd taken out a hefty mortgage to buy a flat and had splashed out on my Jeep. I hadn't gone crazy, but they were things I enjoyed owning and could afford. As I was young and fit, I hadn't bothered with health insurance. That's one mistake I really wish I'd never made. I decided to tackle the biggest problem first and went to see my building society manager.

'The point is,' I said as I sat down in his brand new office in Croydon, south London, 'there's nothing I can do about all of this. I can't help being ill and I can't go back to work until British Airways gives me the all-clear.' He looked at me sympathetically.

'Even if I keep my job I won't be on such good pay as I was when I took out my mortgage. I won't get the allowances for long flights.'

In for a penny, in for a pound I thought. I didn't want to cry but I did feel desperate. I'd never had money troubles before; if I wanted something I bought it. I never gave it a second thought. Those days were over and my God was I missing them. The worst bit was, it was all so unfair. It wasn't my fault that I was in debt.

'Try not to worry too much about this, Carole,' said the manager.

'But I do worry, it's practically all I ever think about.'

'Look, you've been perfectly honest and believe me, that's unusual,' he said. 'A lot of people pile up debts of thousands and thousands before they face the music. At least we all know where we stand. Why don't you pay off your debt a bit at a time, do you think you could manage that?'

'What do you mean? You're not going to repossess my flat?' I could feel my mood lightening for the first time in weeks.

'No, of course not,' he said, smiling. 'Why would we do that? This is a genuine case and you've bothered to tell us what's happening in your life. We don't want to repossess you, we want to help you if we can.'

I couldn't believe what I was hearing. I had walked into this room half an hour earlier assuming I was about to lose my home and now I was being given a chance to keep it. The debt was still there, but I felt a lot better now that the problem was out in the open.

I really resented being on my own through all of this but I had to keep reminding myself that it wasn't Craig's fault that I had MS. Why should he turn his life upside down because I was ill? I spoke to him every other day on the phone, but I didn't want to scare him. Debts, symptoms, job worries, I dealt with them all alone rather than gamble on him leaving me. I didn't really think he would. We were in love, we were inseparable. Craig-and-Carole, our friends joked, it was impossible to think of one without the other. So why was I protecting him from the changes going on in my life? I gave him a call.

'Hi, Craig, how are you doing?' As he answered the phone I could picture exactly where he was standing in the clubhouse in Finland.

'Caz, how's things? I'm missing you. When can you come out here again? Soon?'

I knew he still wasn't reading about MS and I knew he was doing what he loved. The gap between us seemed impossible to bridge.

'I'll see what I can do. I love you.'

I put down the phone and sat in my flat crying and crying. I felt so frightened about everything. Nothing was certain any more. I was drowning in fear. The phone rang: it was my dad.

'Hello, Carole, are you keeping OK?'

'Dad, I don't think I can cope.' My voice cracked as I started to cry again. I knelt on the carpet in my living-room at my wit's end.

'Remember, Carole,' he replied after a pause, 'there are people out there a lot worse off than you.'

'I don't give a shit about anybody else, Dad, what about me?' I shouted. I couldn't believe it! He didn't have a clue what was going on in my life. It wasn't happening to him and as I wasn't telling him how scared I was about my future, how could he possibly understand?

'I don't know what to say.' He sounded upset.

That was the bottom line: what do you say to somebody in my situation? It's not going to go away, and things won't get better. I sat on the floor and leaned back against the sofa. I needed to do some painful thinking.

Was I being honest with people? What was really eating away at me was that I was alone. This illness was the enemy and there was nobody by my side in the battle against it. It was changing me, too. That hadn't been me talking to my dad. I knew he was just trying to help. I felt so angry and hated myself for feeling like that. *I didn't want to be angry.*

In the weeks after my diagnosis I was gradually feeling better and better physically. I was tired but almost all the numbness had gone, except for a patch in the palm of my left hand. I was even driving again. Then British Airways called me in to see their head of health services.

It was strange driving to Heathrow airport out of uniform. The journey was so familiar and yet everything was different for me. I was really nervous. If they took my job away from me ... well, with all the hard truths I'd faced up to in recent weeks, that was one I couldn't bear to think about. I didn't just do my job, I loved my job. But this wasn't like the day I'd gone for my diagnosis. I was facing this alone, hardly anyone knew I had this appointment. It wasn't the old, bubbly, healthy me going to see this doctor. It was the new, private, wary me.

Dr Sandra Mooney was lovely. She had the kindest face and as I sat down in her consulting room in Speedbird House I spotted all my medical notes piled up on one side of her desk. Here we go again, I thought.

'Carole, it's lovely to meet you,' she said. 'I think it's best if we get straight down to business. My most important question first: "What do you want to do?"'

'I want to keep flying,' I said, quick as a flash. 'I love it, it's all I want to do really.' I stopped, feeling a bit embarrassed. No need to overdo it.

'Well, your neurologist – Dr Monro isn't it? She thinks you should keep flying. She feels you've already lost your health, you shouldn't lose your job, too.'

'What do you think, Dr Mooney?' I asked.

'I think you can fly and I think we should play things by ear. Let's see what happens. I want what's best for BA and what's best for you, Carole.'

I felt like kissing her! They didn't see the inevitable wheelchair, I wasn't going to lose my job.

'Now, we're going to put some restrictions on you, Carole,' Dr Mooney explained. 'I'm afraid you won't be on long-haul any longer.'

I'd sort of expected it, but it was still sad. Rio had been my last long-haul job and I hadn't even known it.

'We don't want your sleep pattern affected and I don't want you too far from home again so that it's difficult to get you back,' Dr Mooney said. 'You must avoid jet lag. I feel the long flights will be too much for you.'

The relief was enormous. But short-haul? They were a different crowd, I didn't know any of them.

'How are you feeling at the moment, Carole? Has your numbness gone yet?'

'I'm absolutely fine now,' I lied.

'Good, then we'll put you on office duties and get you booked in for short-haul training, shall we?'

I worked three days a week in the long-haul fleet office as the general dogsbody. It was good to be out working again and it was just in the nick of time. My sick pay was about to run out, I was within a few weeks of going on to no pay at all. But what a difference these few months had made. I was seeing familiar faces every day; it was the office where the cabin crew came in and out all the time, in their uniforms, just off on a flight or just back from somewhere. I watched them with a pang of jealousy. I'd give the manager a nod and nip out to have a cigarette and gossip with them, but already I was moving away from their world. I missed my old job and my old lifestyle so much it was like an ache.

One baking hot day, after I'd been in the office for a few weeks, I was answering a phone call and started to twiddle my pen in my left hand. It was the little bit of numbness I hadn't told Dr Mooney about. As I was talking, I realized I could feel the pen. I twiddled a bit more, then dropped the pen and flexed my hand, open, shut, open, shut. I spread out my fingers as far as they would go. I rested the phone under my chin and prodded my left hand with the fingers of my right hand. I had my whole body back! I was normal again! I finished the phone call quickly and rang Craig's number in Finland.

'Craig, guess what? Guess what's happened,' I whispered down the phone.

'Caz, are you OK? Where are you? Stop whispering.'

'Craig, I'm not numb any more. It's brilliant, I'm normal again!'

'Oh Caz, that's great! I love you. This is great news.'

A week later BA told me I would start flying again in September and put me on a retraining course at Gatwick airport. I'd been flying for two-and-a-half years, but now I was a new girl again. I had to start from scratch on the smaller aircraft, learning where everything was. Something else was different too. I started to feel nervous about my job.

People would expect me to know what I was doing from my first day on short-haul, but I was used to long flights. I'd always had time to chat to the passengers and loads of time to serve meals. Now, on a 40-minute flight from London to Manchester, I still had to serve everyone with tea and coffee and I ended up running around like an idiot.

Still, my first few days back at work were wonderful. As far as other crew knew, I'd chosen to move from long-haul. I was meant to tell my boss on each flight what my problem was, but I didn't bother after the first few flights. I had no symptoms, life was getting back to normal, I almost forgot that I had MS. I felt great after six months off work.

On my fourth night back I arrived home, took off my uniform and noticed that my body felt so heavy it was as though I'd doubled in weight. Even lifting a cup was difficult. I must be tired. It was hardly surprising; I wasn't used to a working week! I read a sloppy postcard from Craig that had been on the doormat. 'I love you and miss you lots,' it said. We'd grown really slushy during this summer apart. I ran a bath and had an early night.

The next morning, my fifth day at work, I had a Glasgow return flight. I was on a break in the crew canteen at lunchtime. I had to wait for a Manchester return trip in the afternoon then I'd have the weekend off. But suddenly my legs and arms began to shake. What was going on? It made me feel panicky. What if someone saw me? Would I get the sack? Should I keep quiet about it? I was afraid that someone at BA, perhaps an executive who didn't even know me, would say: 'We thought you'd cope but we were obviously wrong. Sorry.'

I would have to see the doctor. I felt it was part of the deal; if BA were willing to keep me on the staff then I had to be honest with them. I had, of course, already decided I would never put other crew or passengers in danger and this was my first test. On my way along the corridor to my manager's office I wondered yet again about how honest I needed to be. As my MS was invisible at that time, I could pretend day to day that nothing was wrong. My manager wasn't in her office, but another of the fleet managers was.

'You look pale, Carole. Feeling a bit air sick?' she asked. We both laughed and I told her I wasn't feeling too good. I didn't want to tell her the whole truth because I didn't feel I could trust anyone. So I rang Dr Mooney.

'What's going on, Carole, don't you feel well?' the doctor asked when she came onto the line. I explained what had happened.

'Perhaps you shouldn't be doing these 12-hour days,' she said. 'Go home and rest for a week.'

I drove home, feeling exhausted. My bubble had burst. I wasn't normal and it was no good kidding myself. Multiple sclerosis was taking control and I felt that I had no say in anything any longer. I had thought I could cover it up, pretend it wasn't there. Perhaps I was in denial. I really don't know. But I didn't want to talk about it to anyone.

I rested and went back to work on a restricted eight-hour roster. Lots of people work like that for all sorts of reasons, mostly back problems. But it was a struggle getting used to my new way of life. I didn't have any friends on short-haul and suddenly, at 24, I was with senior staff who wanted short flights for their own reasons – family commitments, that sort of thing. Short-haul, I quickly learned, is a job. Long-haul had been a way of life. But, God, I was lucky to be flying. It got me out of bed every day.

At the end of September, Craig rang me in Vienna where I was on an overnight stop.

'Caz, guess what? I'm coming home.'

'I don't believe it. When?' I screamed down the phone.

'Tomorrow!'

It was heaven for me. I was working six days on, three days off, and coming home every evening to Craig. I was in my element. The difficulties between Craig and me in Finland had just been his way of coping with my diagnosis, I could see that now. This reunion was like a honeymoon, better than ever. I was so glad to have him with me.

But a lot had changed in the six months we'd been apart.

For one thing, I had stopped drinking. I'd learned the hard way that because MS affects my co-ordination, drinking alcohol exaggerated my symptoms. Just before Craig had left for Finland he'd taken me to our favourite Italian restaurant for my birthday. I was enjoying my third glass of red wine when I had to dash to the ladies to throw up. I hadn't had a drink since. I didn't really notice it while he was away, but when he came home he realized he had a driver at his beck and call every time we went out.

I had just come in from work when Craig shouted through to the bathroom where I was changing out of my uniform: 'Hey Caz, let's go into Wimbledon Village for a drink.'

'Not tonight, Craig, if you don't mind. I'm exhausted,' I shouted back. I just wanted to curl up on the sofa and build up my strength for work tomorrow.

'Oh, come on Caz, don't be so boring. You don't mind driving, do you?'

'Yes I do actually. I mind very much,' I shouted back. I could feel my mood changing. I was so tired, why couldn't he understand that? I walked through to the living-room where Craig was sitting.

'Look, Craig, I've just about got enough energy to get through a working day and look after myself. I can't do any more than that. I'm sorry.'

'Going out for a quick drink doesn't seem too much to ask,' he said. But the way I was feeling at that time, it was far too much to ask.

We had a lot of adapting to do in those few months. Bit by bit I filled Craig in with what had been happening while he was away. Now he was home he paid most of the bills and bought the groceries; the mortgage was mine. I thought I was getting back on my feet financially when a letter came saying the hire purchase company was about to repossess my lovely Jeep. I adored that car. But I was £900 in arrears. I was crying over the letter when Craig came home one evening.

'They're going to take my Jeep away, Craig,' I said, keeping my cool but wishing he could wave a magic wand.

'Don't worry, Caz,' he replied, 'that won't happen.'

He made me want to scream. 'It's about to happen any day, here's the proof!' I waved the letter at him.

'OK, if it means that much to you I'll pay the bill,' he said after he'd read through the letter several times.

He'd given me a reprieve and I loved him for it. I didn't know then that within a few months I'd be selling the Jeep to pay off other debts. Sometimes it's just as well we don't know the full picture.

Craig and I had always had a traditional relationship, I suppose. I cooked, washed up, all that stuff, and kept the flat clean. Now I was finding I couldn't do it all.

'I know this is difficult, but you've got to pull your weight from now on,' I said to him one evening. I'd just come in from work and found a pile of dirty dishes in the sink. A few months before, I wouldn't have batted an eyelid. Now it made me so angry I wished I was three years old; I wanted to be able to lie on the floor and kick and scream and cry till I was sick. Life was so damned hard these days.

'I will, Caz, I promise,' he said and on the whole he did. But it was dawning on me that the one thing we never discussed was multiple sclerosis. Why didn't I just say to him: 'Look, I'm ill and I can't do everything any more?' Was I afraid of losing him?

I began to get a different perspective on life in the months after my diagnosis. If something was important to me, it became a big issue. And babies had always been important to me. I'd spent four years as a nanny before training as a stewardess and had always planned to have a family of my own. Friends would often leave their kids with me. 'You don't mind, Carole, do you? We know how much you love them.' It was true.

One night lying in bed the words of Ashley, the counsellor on the day I'd been diagnosed, came into my head. I'd kept my job and sex wasn't a problem, I thought, as I remembered the three questions I had asked her. But what about children? 'Try to have a baby earlier rather than later,' she'd said. 'Giving birth can trigger a relapse.' Her words suddenly made me panic.

'Craig, don't you think it would be a good idea if we had a baby?' I said to him as we snuggled up under the duvet.

'Of course it is, Caz, but not right now,' he said. 'There's too much going on, we don't know what's going to happen next.'

Craig knew I loved babies, but he didn't know that waves of panic were sweeping over me every time I wondered when the next relapse would be. There was a silence.

'The point is, Caz, we've got plenty of time to have kids later. We should wait till I've finished working in Finland. It makes more sense to think about this when I'm here all year round.'

I didn't want to push him away but I wanted marriage and a family, and I wanted them now. There might not be a 'later'. I could feel myself starting to panic again. Damn this MS, I thought, but I didn't tell Craig that. In fact, there was a lot I wasn't telling him at that time.

Craig's mum lived in South Africa and we flew off to visit her in Johannesburg for three weeks in the autumn. I spent long days sitting in the sun and my tan turned a lovely deep brown, a shade I hadn't managed since giving up long-haul flights. I did feel a pang of guilt when I thought of Dr Fritz in Rio telling me not to sunbathe, but that was months ago. Nobody had mentioned it since so I decided that ignorance is bliss. One evening the three of us went out to dinner.

'Caz and I were talking about getting married, Mum,' Craig said out of the blue. I looked up, surprised that my hints had filtered through to him.

His mum had always liked me but she didn't say anything for a while. 'What *do* you mean?' she said, looking straight at her son as if he'd gone mad.

An atmosphere spread around the table. Anne is a nursing sister and the last thing she wanted for her son was to see him looking after a sick wife for years on end. As his mother, she must have thought that was the wrong way round. She wanted a wife for Craig who would care for him. Later, when the two of them were alone, she pointed out that as a golf pro he could earn a fortune in Johannesburg.

'If you come here to work you're on your own,' I told him when he mentioned it to me. I didn't like the city, it made me feel as though I was living in a fortress. But I knew that wasn't the point. I'd been taught another hard lesson. I wasn't just Carole any more, I was Carole with MS and that must have been hard for her to accept. She was obviously concerned about our future.

My tan was just fading when I came home one night to find Craig and his brother, Colin, watching football on TV. As I walked through the door, the phone rang. It was my mum in Australia. Doug, my gorgeous, handsome, lovely cousin, had died from a drugs overdose. Mum and I couldn't think of anything to say to each other, the news was too shocking for words.

'How could Doug do that? How dare he put the family through this?' I shouted at no-one in particular. There was no reply from the pair on the sofa.

I burst into tears and the brothers looked at each other. They moved up to make room for me on the sofa and I sat next to Craig. He put his arms around me and gave me a hug. But he carried on watching the football match.

We didn't say anything. What was there to say? Craig didn't understand what I was feeling. Couldn't he see how hard it was for me to keep myself together? How could Doug have been so selfish? I would never see him again and that really hurt. I didn't say any more, though. I expected Craig to understand everything. After a while I went to bed, exhausted with thinking. As it turned out, Doug's overdose had been accidental, not suicide. It happened just over a year after his father had died from a heart attack.

I knew in my head that I was ill but I didn't let it show. As my body was behaving itself it became easier and easier for me to pretend that everything was fine again. I didn't want to go to meetings with other people with MS. I wouldn't be able to cope with seeing them, I wasn't ready for all of that. Of course, what I really didn't want was to see what the disease can do to you. What if there were people at those meetings in more advanced stages of the illness? I felt happier pretending.

It was no coincidence that Craig and I spent the New Year with my grandparents, Peter and Annie Crawford. They were the only people I hadn't told about my illness. They were both in their eighties and wouldn't have understood multiple sclerosis. It would have devastated them. As far as they were concerned I was happy, healthy and with the man I loved. That's all I wanted them to see.

We arrived at their little end-of-terrace house in Banff, Scotland, and there they were standing on the doorstep waiting as Craig and I struggled out of the car, balancing our late Christmas presents and trying to shut the car doors without dropping anything. The cold went right into my bones and Grandad showed us in to sit by the fire.

'It's good to have you home, my darling,' he said sitting down next to me and holding my hand, his bright blue eyes sparkling. He was always happiest with his family around him and my sister and I were the apple of his eye. We had spent most of our childhood days living round the corner from them. While Mum and Dad were at work, my grandparents had looked after us. For years I was Grandad's shadow. I even had a pair of overalls to wear when I was little because I wanted to look like him.

As Grandad and I sat hand in hand, memories came flooding back. Nowhere else felt quite so safe as their house, nowhere else even smelt like it, that homely smell of a real fire. This was home to me. But right now it was late and Craig and I went to bed. Grandma came up to tuck us in. We might be in our twenties and living together, but I was still her little Carole.

'I love you, my darling,' she said leaning over to kiss me goodnight. 'It's good to have you both here. Sleep tight.'

I had made the right decision I thought as I drifted off to sleep. I was living a lie, but white lies can be a good thing. They really didn't need to know that I was ill.

That New Year was one of the best in my life. Multiple sclerosis seemed a long way away as we all made our way to the Central Bar in Banff on New Year's Eve. We'd left Grandad and Grandma at home, but the rest of the family braved the biting cold. After a piper piped in 1992 the owners, friends who had grown up in Banff with my parents, shut the doors and threw a party. Outside, hailstones lashed at the windows and later, as Craig and I walked home through the streets in the early hours of the morning, my fingers and toes ached with the cold. But I felt truly happy.

We spent New Year's Day with my grandparents and went for a meal at a restaurant overlooking Macduff harbour. Grandad, smart in a grey suit and navy blue tie, sat opposite me.

'Grandad, do you remember the spider?'

'Of course I do, my darling. How old would she have been then, Annie?' He turned to my grandma next to him. This was a favourite family story. It was lovely to sit looking out at the sea listening to it being told again.

'You were a wee thing, about five I think,' Grandma said, smiling.

'You had insisted that we gave you a pair of my overalls, so that you looked like me,' Grandad said, in his stride by now. 'I fixed a hook in the garage for them to hang on. One morning, you wanted to help me clean my car. I got you into your overalls and rolled up the legs and sleeves – they were far too big for you. I was putting mine on when you let out a scream. I can hear it now. I turned back and you had your arm out in front of you with your little hand spread wide open and a spider crawling across it. You were terrified!'

'I remember you slapping my hand to get the spider off,' I said. 'It must have crept out of the overalls. That slap really hurt! I still hate spiders.'

'You never went into the garage again, either,' Grandad added. 'I had to bring the car out onto the driveway if you were going to help me. Now, Carole, which cutlery do I use for this?' He looked at me, grinning innocently as he cut into his ice-cream with a knife and fork.

'What on earth are you doing, Grandad, you silly billy?' I said, pretending to be outraged. He was at his best playing the fool for us.

'Carole,' my Grandad said to me in the car on the way home, 'I do wish that I could see more of you and your sister.'

'I wish that too, Grandad,' I said, giving him a hug.

'You know how much I love you, don't you, my darling? Happy New Year. Let's hope this will be a good one for all of us.'

Craig and I left for England and home the next day. As we drove away, I turned round in my seat and saw my grandparents arm-in-arm at their doorway. Married for more than 60 years, they really were a couple so in love that I couldn't imagine them apart. I wound down the car window.

'I'll be back soon, Grandad, don't worry. I promise,' I shouted out across the cold air. He waved and smiled and was just turning back into his front door as the car turned the corner.

5. Starting to Panic

Please God, don't let me collapse, not now. I looked up at the sky, grey and empty, and down at the tiny figure of my Grandma as the coffin was lowered into its grave. That can't be my Grandad in there, I thought. I put my arm around grandma's shoulders. She seemed so frail. How on earth was she going to survive on her own? This was the first funeral I'd had to deal with and I felt frightened. Grandma didn't know I had multiple sclerosis and I was aware that a shock like this could trigger a relapse. I was determined she wouldn't see that happen.

I had known Grandad was ill at the beginning of March. It was just a week before that I had booked a car to take me off a flight to Aberdeen straight to the hospital. But I'd been stuck in Madrid when something went wrong with the aircraft and I hadn't made it. He had died and I hadn't been there.

By the time Craig and I arrived in Banff Grandma's little house was filled with people standing around looking shocked, not quite knowing what to do. I still hadn't cried but all the time, inside my head, there was a picture of Grandad, my Grandad. It was only three months since we'd been chatting and laughing over dinner on New Year's Day. Now I would never see him again.

'Carole, would you like to see him?' Auntie Angela asked. 'He's in the chapel of rest.'

I wasn't expecting a building site. The chapel was still being built and we had to step over rubble and along planks of wood to reach it. Uncle Peter had the key and I stared at the door, not wanting to go in, not wanting to accept that Grandad was dead.

'You'll be fine, Carole, he looks very peaceful,' my uncle said gently. Craig stood behind me and Auntie Angela held my arm. We had to climb over the threshold because the steps hadn't yet been put in place and we all clambered into a freezing cold room, just breeze block walls not yet plastered. Alone in the centre was a coffin resting on two builders' trestles.

I can't describe the sound that came from my mouth as I realized where we were, what we were doing. It was a howl of pure grief and it echoed around that hollow room. Everything was blurred and I stretched out my hand to touch Grandad. I wanted to wake him up but he was cold and as I looked down my hand went into spasm. Then, at last, the tears started to come. My auntie – who had lost her husband, her son and now her father within 18 months – began to sob quietly behind me. But she took the note I had written for Grandad and a little teddy bear I'd bought and placed them in the coffin.

We left the room and I looked out across the sea. I felt so embarrassed by what I'd done, howling, collapsing in tears, making a spectacle of myself.

'Don't worry, Carole, it's perfectly normal,' my auntie said in the car on the way home. I hated the fact that Craig had seen it all.

By the day of the funeral I was terrified I would have a relapse. I kept thinking that this shock would put me in a wheelchair. My family were concerned, too. I wanted my mum but I was glad she hadn't come over from Australia. Watching her grief at losing her father would have been too much for me. I was pulling on my black boots in the bedroom when somebody called up the stairs.

'Carole, the hearse is just coming up the street. We've got to hurry.'

The church, Our Lady of Mount Carmel, is old and small. I walked in and was surprised that it was packed with people – and horrified at the sight of the coffin in front of the altar. I felt shaky and weak and the service seemed to go on for ever. When the piper began 'Amazing Grace' all I could see was Grandad's face. I'd sung the song as a solo in a school concert when I was 10 and Grandad had been in the audience, beaming with pride and giving me the thumbs-up sign each time he caught my eye. My sister Hazel moved towards me as she noticed the look on my face. 'I thought you were going to pass out,' she told me afterwards. But I didn't.

After the burial, we turned away from the graveside and walked up the winding path to the entrance gate. I was tired with grief and with the effort of keeping myself together in front of everyone. Craig put his arm around me.

'Are you all right, Caz?' he asked.

'Of course I'm not all right! What a stupid question!' I shouldn't have said that. Poor Craig, he'd been through enough in the last few days.

We both had to go back to work and were due to fly from Aberdeen to London the next day. When we reached the airport, though, a plane had overshot the runway and it was closed. We were all put on a coach to Edinburgh for a flight from there. I sat back in my seat and closed my eyes. I didn't want to speak to anyone and I didn't have the energy to make polite conversation. Then 'Amazing Grace' came over the coach radio.

'Craig, tell the driver to switch that off.'

'It'll be over soon, honey.'

'Please do it, now! I can't stand it.'

Craig went up to the front of the coach and a few seconds later there was silence as the radio clicked off.

'Thank you, Craig. I'm sorry,' I said as he came back to his seat. He didn't say anything and I closed my eyes again.

Back in London all I really wanted to do was work. Instead I was signed off for three weeks of complete rest. I felt empty and exhausted. Alone in the flat during the day, I cried and cried. My legs were tingling but I chose to ignore that. Then I started to notice a feeling of butterflies in my stomach, a fear that something awful was about to happen.

I began to wonder what would happen next, what would I lose? What if Craig died? What would I do then? I worried that my grandfather might have thought I'd let him down by not being with him when he died. I was dealing, suddenly, with lots of different emotions which I couldn't talk about to anybody. And at the back of my mind all the time was the fear that I might have a relapse.

Craig, on the other hand, couldn't have been happier. He had only a few more weeks before he could go back to Finland for another glorious summer of golf, golf and golf. He would burst into the flat after work, read a newspaper, watch TV, completely content in his own world. He couldn't see the anger building up inside me. He didn't notice that I was falling apart. I watched in amazement as our worlds drifted further and further away from each other. It made me want to punch him so that he could feel some of the hurt, have some understanding of how I was feeling.

'Craig, why don't you try to understand me?' I asked him one evening when the anger inside me felt ready to explode. I needed to have an argument.

'How can I understand, Caz?'

'You could try talking to me,' I screamed. 'Or is that too much to ask?'

'How can I understand what you're going through when nobody close to me has ever died, Caz? Be fair.'

He was missing the point and I couldn't even make him see what that point was. I wasn't just grieving for my grandfather, although that was bad enough. I was grieving the loss of my health, how short life was, how uncertain my future looked, how frightened I was.

I stormed out of the flat. It was the only way I knew of not attacking him. I put a tape in my car cassette player and drove round and round the streets. I parked and rested my head on the steering wheel, sobbing. Why me? Why does everything bad have to happen to me? I've only just had my twenty-fourth birthday. Give me a break, for God's sake. Eventually I grew calm again and I drove home.

I was back at work by the time Craig went to Finland in April. I missed him desperately but it was different this time. The separation made me feel angry as well as lonely. Then a new manager was appointed and I felt very nervous when she asked to see me. Now what's going to go wrong for me?

'I've been told your situation, Carole,' Maggie Sheppard said on our first meeting in her office at Heathrow. 'I don't want you to worry about your sickness. If you're ill, go home and rest and forget all about us.'

'I do worry, though,' I replied.

'Look at it this way, Carole. I'd rather you rested and came back to us soon than had a relapse and had to be away for six months.'

I felt that I could trust Maggie implicitly. A little later I had the chance of a five-day week with no weekend work. I leapt at it. At last I could fit in with friends at home who were in normal jobs. At least things were looking up on the work front.

It was on one of my first proper weekends at home that I had my first panic attack. I was in the back seat of a friend's car when I realized it had no back passenger doors. I was trapped!

'Can you stop the car, please,' I heard myself saying. Then loudly: 'Stop the car, now!'

My friend pulled in to the side of the road and I felt a wave of relief as I climbed out of the car and walked round and round, trying to gulp in fresh air and get my breathing back to normal.

'Sorry, everyone. Just humour me.' I managed a smile when I saw how concerned my friends were looking. But I was shaking with fear and as I settled into the front passenger seat I wound down the window, still needing to feel fresh air on my face. As we set off I couldn't believe what I'd done.

A few days later I was in a packed lift and the same thing happened. I stopped the lift on the next floor and pushed my way out. As I walked the rest of the way up the stairs I suddenly thought: 'My God, what if this happens when I'm in an aircraft? I'll lose my job.' It was time to see my doctor.

'So what you're saying is, I need to see a shrink?' I looked at the doctor in disbelief. I'd asked her for an explanation of my panic attacks and instead she was writing down a name for me on a slip of paper.

'We prefer to call them psychologists, Carole,' she said smiling at me. 'This one's very good. I think she'll be able to help you.'

Dr Susan Mumford, principal clinical psychologist, was wearing a huge silver ring which rattled every time she moved her hand. It distracted me as I sat waiting for her to begin whatever it is that psychologists do. I didn't like her or her gloomy office at St George's Hospital in Tooting.

'Tell me about your illness, Carole,' she started.

'It doesn't bother me at all,' I answered, wishing I'd never agreed to this sort of investigation.

'Your doctor tells me that your grandfather has died recently. Would you like to talk about that?'

'I miss him,' I replied. 'But I'd expect to. He was important to me.'

'And why was that? Tell me something about your background.'

She was making me feel angry with her prying questions, but I plodded on. As we spoke I found myself wondering what she could teach me about my situation. After a bad start, I began to listen and felt surprised that certain things were falling into place.

'Carole, from what you've been telling me you don't seem to have cried much recently but you are angry.'

'I cry when I'm on my own, but never in front of anyone else.'

'It could be that you feel more in control when you're angry. Letting someone else see you cry would take away your control. Does that make sense?'

'But I don't want to be an angry person. I don't want to be angry with Craig all the time.'

'You have to remember that being diagnosed with multiple sclerosis has made you feel you no longer have control over your own life. I think that loss is what has brought on your panic attacks.'

'I don't see how being ill could do that,' I said.

'The attacks are your way of trying to regain control. So, if you're in a vulnerable position you feel you have to take action – like getting out of the lift.' I considered what she was saying.

'OK, I can see that makes sense,' I said. 'But what can I do about it?'

Dr Mumford taught me to clear my mind if I felt an attack coming so that I could concentrate on my breathing pattern. She suggested I might look into meditation – and then she told me to cry more.

'You must not be afraid to cry, Carole,' she said. 'When you see

Craig again talk to him about it. Ask him to say to you "You're obviously upset" when you start to argue and then let you cry your eyes out. There's no need to let him feel you're not in control. Crying doesn't make you weak, it means you're doing yourself a lot of good.'

'But I feel embarrassed when I'm crying.'

'Please try it, Carole, whatever it is that you're feeling must come out. The only other thing feelings can do is to fester. And when I see you next we'll go in a lift together so that I can show you some practical things you can do to avoid panicking.'

I had been with Dr Mumford for two hours and for once I was glad to be going home to an empty flat. I made a pot of coffee, lit a Silk Cut cigarette and mulled over everything she had told me.

She was spot on about my anger. It was making me tired. I didn't want to be angry, it wasn't as though I liked what I had become. I hated needing to see a psychologist, but I was glad I had seen her. It wasn't something you heard people talking about a lot. I suppose nobody's proud of it so nobody likes to admit to it. My MS wasn't going to go away but I didn't really know what to do with it. It *had* taken control of my life, but I didn't know how I was meant to stop that. It wasn't just the MS, though. The bottom line was that if I stayed angry I would lose Craig and that would be the one thing that I couldn't bear. Thoughts, thoughts, thoughts. If only I could switch off my mind and have a rest.

Dr Mumford had made a lot of sense about losing control. I decided not to see her again, though. I had learnt as much as I needed from her. Much later, I phoned Craig.

'I've been to see the psychologist,' I said, nervous and still slightly embarrassed even though he knew about my appointment with her.

'Did you? What happened?'

'She told me that I need to stop being so angry and one way of helping that is that I should cry more.'

'Well, what can I do about that?'

'If I start to get angry with you, it could just be that I'm upset. We need to find out why I'm upset, get to the bottom of it.'

'All right, Caz, whatever you say.'

If people had known the black thoughts going on in my head at that time they'd have been shocked. Instead, every day I was putting on my uniform, driving to Heathrow and reporting for duty with a smile. It was a strange time: I was settling in on short-haul but I wasn't talking about my illness. If someone wanted to know why I'd left long-haul I'd just say: 'Oh, my body couldn't take it.' If they pressed me on how I'd managed a transfer to short-haul, my stock reply was: 'I was diagnosed with multiple sclerosis. But I'm fine.' It was *my* illness. I didn't need to talk about it to everyone and I didn't want to be 'Carole Mackie, you know, the one with MS'. I just wanted to get on with my job.

But the MS was there, as it kept reminding me. There'd be a patch of numbness somewhere, or a tingling sensation, often in my feet. Then I would panic and throw myself into work to take my mind off it, which in turn made me exhausted. I was in a classic situation. I wasn't listening to my body because mentally I needed my job. I thought I'd be all right all the time and I just kept working and leading what I thought was a normal life. I wasn't aware that these symptoms were warning me to rest.

A few weeks after I saw the psychologist I was put on a standard return flight to Oslo in Norway. As I was serving lunch I felt a pain in my ears. By the end of the flight I was in such agony that as soon as the last passenger had gone I asked for a nurse. Within minutes one came on to the plane.

'I'm sorry, Carole, but I can't let you fly with this infection,' she told me. I was angry but there was nothing I could do. I booked into the crew hotel, the Plaza, collapsed into bed – and didn't move for three days. I spoke to Craig on the phone each day and other crew popped in to see if I was OK. One of the managers at Heathrow called me.

'Now Carole, you're sure this isn't the MS?' he asked, concerned that I was having a relapse.

'It's an ear infection,' I said. 'It could happen to anyone.'

On the fourth day I had to visit the BA doctor in Oslo for another examination and he grounded me. I came out of his surgery and hailed a taxi.

'What's the matter, you look unhappy,' the lady taxi driver said as she looked in her rear-view mirror at me.

'Oh, it's nothing, I've just got an ear infection so I'm grounded. I'm an air stewardess,' I said. There was a short silence.

'Did you know Michael Jackson's in concert here tomorrow night?'

'You're kidding. I'm a real fan.'

'You should get a ticket. It might cheer you up.'

'No, I really don't feel up to it.'

That evening I went down to the hotel restaurant for dinner. It was time for a change of scenery. The restaurant was busy. I sat alone at a table for two and ordered a glass of Diet Coke.

'Do you mind if we join you?'

I looked up and saw two men and a woman, all beautifully dressed.

'Of course, please do,' I said and they sat on the adjoining table. I introduced myself.

'Your English is very good,' said the one who had told me his name was Bruno Taco Falcon.

'It should be!' I laughed. 'I'm Scottish, actually, but I live in England.'

'Oh, sorry,' said the girl, Yuko Sumida Holley. 'It's your blonde hair and blue eyes. We assumed you were Norwegian.'

I told them I was a stewardess but had been grounded and the third, Lavelle Smith, said: 'I'm ill, too. I've got a terrible sore throat.'

I rummaged around in my bag and found some throat lozenges.

'Try these, they're really good,' I said.

They were great fun and during the meal they told me that they were Michael Jackson's dancers. Others joined us and we all drifted to the bar, where there was more room. I couldn't believe my luck when one of them gave me an all-access pass to the concert.

'This lets you sit at the back near the dancers' dressing room,' he said. 'You can just nip out if you don't feel well. Come early, we'll show you around.'

When I reached the stadium Yuko still had her rollers in. I couldn't recognize the men in their full make-up. The atmosphere backstage was incredibly relaxed and friendly; it was hard to believe they were about to perform in front of thousands of people. When the support artist, Rozalla, started to rehearse and 'Everybody's Free' came blasting from the speakers we all danced along the corridor outside the dressing-rooms. Goodness knows what we looked like but we were laughing so much that we didn't care. Then I found my seat, on a balcony to the side of the stage, right at the front. What a brilliant view!

As I looked across the stage, I could see Michael Jackson's stretch limousine arriving quietly at a back entrance. And it was a strange thing, but throughout the concert I didn't watch the star. As Michael Jackson leapt onto the stage I found myself looking out for Taco, Lavelle and Yuko. Where were they? Oh, there they were – larger than life – and I'd been chatting to them a few hours before. I knew this was something I would never forget.

After the concert Lavelle came and found me with a beer. 'Here you are, Carole. What did you think of the show?'

'For once in my life, I'm almost speechless. It was unbelievable! You were all brilliant! I just loved it.'

He grinned. 'Sounds like you enjoyed it. I'm glad.'

For a whole day multiple sclerosis had disappeared from my mind. Everyone had been so kind to me. I felt better, absolutely normal again. It was a great way to be.

Within a week I was back in another honeymoon period. It was September and Craig came home from Finland, that first excitement of being together again running high. We went to a friend's party, and although I felt tired I couldn't resist having a dance. I could see Craig sitting on the floor with his back against the wall, chatting to someone. I had been dancing for a few minutes when I realized something was very wrong. My legs felt heavy, as if someone had put bricks in my shoes. I couldn't do it.

'Craig, I feel like an old woman,' I said, sliding down the wall to sit next to him. He rubbed my leg.

'No you don't, honey,' he said.

I wanted to yell at him: 'Yes I do, why can't you just accept that?'

I wanted him to put his arms around me so that I could sob away all this anger and hurt. But he didn't. So I couldn't.

Three weeks later a big patch of my leg behind my right knee went numb. I was scared, really scared, and went to see my doctor.

'What shall I do?' I asked the locum when my name was called. 'I'm meant to be going on a three-day trip to Tel Aviv. I know I can't be stuck out there if I'm taken ill, but the trip's worth £100.'

'Rubbish, Carole,' he replied. 'This could be a relapse. There's no question about it, you can't go. You must rest.'

The numbness lasted three weeks and with it came an over-whelming tiredness. I'd had so many warning signs and ignored them. Now I was paying the price. But these weeks off work here and there were beginning to add up, and every time I was off I lost more money.

'Caz, how much have you lost being off work this time?' Craig asked me one night as we were sitting at home.

'What does it matter?' I screamed. Of all the questions he could have been asking me, was that really all he could think about?

'I was just wondering, that's all.'

'Don't make this situation worse than it already is, Craig.'

'Caz, you're obviously upset, honey.'

'Don't patronize me!'

He grinned. As I burst into tears we both realized what he had done. Craig had taken the psychologist's advice, he had said exactly what she had suggested. And it had worked.

'I can't stand it, Craig, I can't bear losing so much money. I'm always in debt.' I cried and cried.

But we still weren't talking about multiple sclerosis.

I went back to work feeling more rested this time. So much so that one night after I had come off a flight and was driving home I phoned Craig and said I'd be late. I wanted to see a friend I hadn't caught up with for ages.

'Come home now, Caz, please.'

'Why? Are you missing me that much?' I joked. But there was something in his voice: I went straight home.

'I've just heard that I can't go back to Finland next year, Caz. They've found a local golf pro to take my place.'

My heart skipped a beat. This was perfect for me; at last he wouldn't be disappearing for six months every year. Then I felt guilty. One look at Craig's face showed me how upset he was. For him, this was a real crisis.

'What am I going to do, Caz? I love it in Finland. I can't stand the winter here if I haven't got the thought of Finland to keep me going.'

He'd left Finland only a few weeks before on the understanding that he'd be going back for another six months the following summer. For the months he wasn't in Finland, Craig did the most boring job you could imagine: packing cartons in the warehouse where his brother was the manager, in fact where we'd met. He'd found it impossible to find a golfing job in Britain that left him with the freedom to spend each summer away.

'Don't worry, Craig, we'll find you a job here, I promise. Even if it means we have to move, that's fine by me.' I didn't really want to move, but here was my chance to help Craig, instead of looking to him for support.

The next few weeks we drove all over Kent, Sussex and Surrey on my weekends off, looking at golf courses and making inquiries about jobs. Craig was still devastated, but at least we were doing something together that was for us as a couple. When I flew off on a night-stop to Barcelona I was feeling really good.

The next morning as I woke up in my hotel in Spain I realized that my eyes ached. I didn't understand why, as I'd had a really long night's sleep – something I was beginning to learn was vital for me now. On the flight home moving my eyes from left to right was painful. Imagine how it felt, walking up and down the aisle looking at passengers. Every movement made me wince. There were shadows developing at the sides of both eyes, too. My eyesight was narrowing down to tunnel vision.

I told the purser but carried on with my job, smiling and worrying. By the time I was driving home the pain was unbearable. I couldn't move my eyes in any direction without feeling that someone was tugging on the nerves behind my eyeballs. There were tiny, sharp pains running down both sides of my face, too.

'Hi, Caz. How are you? Was the flight good?' Craig looked up as I walked into the flat.

'I'm a bit tired. I think I'll have a bath,' was all I said.

He popped out to the shops and I lay in the bath feeling a fear that was close to panic. Not blindness, please God, don't let me go blind. I could think of nothing else. I was so weak that when I got out of the bath I wrapped a towel around myself and, without bothering to rub myself dry, I literally crawled on all fours to the bedroom.

'What's up, honey?' Craig said when he came back home to find me sprawled across the bed, still wrapped in the bath towel.

'I don't feel very well, I can't move my eyes properly,' I said, and started to cry. 'I need to see the doctor.'

I went to the surgery in pyjamas with my coat over the top. Craig sat next to me in the waiting-room. I was so weary that all I wanted to do was stretch out on the chairs and sleep. It took every ounce of self-control to remain upright in my seat. At last my name was called.

'Are you coming in with me, Craig?' I asked.

'No, Caz, I'll wait out here.' I walked into the surgery.

'Now Carole,' the doctor said, 'I want you to follow this pen with your eyes.' He took a Biro from his breast pocket and passed it in front of my face. I put my head in my hands and leant on the doctor's desk.

'I'm sorry, I just can't. They hurt too much.' I started to cry again.

'You poor little sausage,' he said. I was so surprised I almost wanted to laugh. I probably would have laughed but by now even speaking made my eyes hurt more. But I'd never been called a little sausage before. Then he told me I'd have to go back to the neurologist at Atkinson Morley Hospital for a proper examination.

That night I had the urge to go to the loo time and time again, but nothing ever happened when I got there. I was exhausted but kept waking and having to dash to the toilet. Each time I grew more and more scared. What the hell was going on? And what would be the next thing to give out? My body was letting me down in ways I'd never even thought about before. It was as though it didn't belong to me any more.

The next morning Craig went off to work and I set out for the hospital alone. At least this time I didn't have to wait months for an appointment so I suppose I was an emergency. My first shock was when the neurologist pointed me towards a bed on a ward.

'I'm not *staying* here,' I said to him, and I could hear the edge of panic in my voice. 'I've only come for some tests.'

But for the time being he only wanted to examine me. By now, the reflex tests were becoming familiar. They always made me think of Dr Fritz in Rio and the first time I'd had them. I told the neurologist about my useless trips to the toilet all through the night, too. He gave me a reassuring smile and walked away from my bed. I could see him talking to a nurse and she smiled, too, as she walked towards me.

'Carole,' she said, 'I need to fit you with a catheter. We need to drain your bladder.'

I couldn't believe what was happening. I was helpless. I'd have to go through with it, it was just that I hadn't been prepared for all this. The nurse set up some equipment by the side of my bed and drew the screens around. As she started to fit the catheter she talked quietly to me.

'God, I don't envy you your job,' I said and laughed. 'Fancy having to stick tubes into people like this. Yuk!'

She was laughing too, but as she looked down and concentrated on her task I began to cry. Just tears, no noise. What could be worse than this? I found it so degrading. It was uncomfortable, it hurt, and I felt embarrassed that this young girl, about my age, had to do this to me. I felt ill and scared. I was already terrified about my eyes, now this. I'd never dreamt this would happen. The nurse looked up and fell silent.

At last it was over. I felt slightly more comfortable but much more upset than when I'd arrived here. I lay back and closed my aching eyes. Was this it, then? The big relapse?

The neurologist came back a little later. 'You're not incontinent, Carole, we've carried out all the tests. But I'm afraid we need to keep you in.'

What! *Incontinent*? Of course I wasn't incontinent. I was a young air stewardess. I'd been at work yesterday, serving passengers with their meals and smiling. People like me aren't incontinent.

'I don't want to stay,' I said much more assertively than I felt.

'You're having a relapse, Carole. We really must monitor you. The only other thing we can do is to give you steroids at this stage.'

'No way!' I exploded. 'I am not taking steroids. What about the side-effects? They make you swell up. They can give you acne. No thank you! And I'm not staying here!'

'It really would be for the best, Carole.'

'Well, actually, I can't stay. Someone's coming to pick me up,' I lied.

I hate hospitals, they make me feel ill. I needed to get out of there as quickly as I could. I climbed down off the bed feeling wobbly and very sore, put my clothes back on and went home.

Craig had been at his packing job, another ordinary day, while I'd been having a catheter fitted. But I wasn't going to tell him that. The indignity of it was still smarting without my boyfriend knowing. How can you discuss incontinence with the man you sleep with? He'd never feel the same way about me again. I kept it all to myself. The alternative, I realized, was to fall apart.

'I'm off work, Craig,' I said when he came in later that day. 'They think I'm having a relapse.'

6. Desperate for Answers

'Well, Craig, yes or no?' I said as I arrived home from work. It felt good to be back in the real world after my six-week relapse. Now the icing on the cake: after travelling hundreds of miles searching for a golf pro vacancy, Craig had been for an interview at a club in Carshalton, Surrey, 10 minutes' drive from our flat. But I couldn't tell from his face which way the interview had gone.

'It's yes, Caz. I got the job.'

I gave a squeal and flung my arms around him. I started to jump up and down, dancing around the flat. This was perfect, at last we'd have some stability. It was our big chance to have a proper relationship.

'Craig, this is the best news ever! We can be together and you'll be golfing. I can't believe it!'

'It's great, Caz,' he said.

'Oh, Craig, look happy! Let's go out to celebrate.'

But when I looked at him I could see there was something missing.

'I'm relieved to have a job, Caz,' was all he said.

Craig threw himself into his new job and I became a regular at his club, meeting him for lunch, sometimes even knocking a few golf balls around. It was important for him to spend time with his clients. A pro relies on word-of-mouth; once you're known, clients will recommend you to their friends and colleagues. My sister, Hazel, finished her nannying job in Switzerland and moved to London, too, so for the first time I had a member of my family living nearby. Then my mum rang from Australia.

'I'm coming over for a visit,' she said. 'I'm bringing Grandma back. It was a good idea to have her out here after Grandad died but she's homesick for Scotland.'

I was in heaven. I'd have Craig, Hazel and my mum around me. I hadn't seen Mum for two years, the longest we'd ever been apart. It was too big a gap. Dropping in on her in Perth was the thing I missed most about long-haul flying. The last time I'd seen her I had been fit and healthy, little knowing what was in store for me. It struck me how much I'd been through since then; falling ill in Rio, being diagnosed with MS. It was like looking back at a different person. I wondered what she would make of me now. I couldn't wait to see her again.

Then I fell ill again.

I'd had tingling in my legs and buzzing down my neck and back for some time but had managed to ignore it. My legs felt really heavy, too, and the week before Mum was due to arrive my doctor signed me off work for three weeks. The one good thing about these symptoms was that I could cover them up. Nobody needed to know what was going on. I could pretend everything was fine. I was determined that Mum would see me looking well and Grandma must never know I was ill.

My plan worked until we went to Scotland and Mum asked me to go with her to Grandad's grave. It would be a first visit for both of us and I didn't really feel ready, let alone well enough, to face it. What if I ended up collapsing at the graveside? It wasn't something my mum needed to see.

'I don't want to go alone, Carole,' Mum said. 'Will you come with me?'

'I'm not really ready yet, Mum,' I answered. 'I'm sorry.'

'Don't worry, darling, I understand,' she said.

I felt so selfish, but the alternative was to tell her the whole truth and I certainly wasn't ready for that. She knew I had MS, she didn't need the details.

We came home to London once Grandma was settled in Scotland and Craig and I had Mum to ourselves. I'd forgotten how much she adored Craig. She really trusted him and seemed to bring out the best in him. Out shopping one day, he disappeared for a while and came back with a bouquet of red roses for me.

'Ah, he's so sweet,' Mum said. And I thought so, too.

By about eight o'clock that evening I was too tired to pretend any longer. I snuggled up to Craig on the sofa and started to doze. Mum leant over the back of the sofa and stroked my face.

'Are you tired, darling?' she said. 'Why don't you go to bed and get some sleep?'

I knew then that she understood. She knew something of what I was going through, and she'd said exactly the right thing. I fell into bed feeling guilty at breaking up the evening, but relieved that I could just rest without having to explain myself. It was good having Mum around.

I was standing in the hallway on the morning Mum was due to fly back to Australia when I heard Craig say: 'OK, Issy, have a good trip.'

'Look after Carole for me, won't you Craig?' she answered, and I could see through the living-room door that she was giving him a hug. How I hated these goodbyes.

'Of course. Don't worry,' he told her.

'I know you will, Craig. I'm so glad she's got you.'

After taking her to the airport, I came home to an empty flat. I sat down in the silence and thought. Should I have spoken to her about my illness? I had said nothing to her about it in the two weeks we'd had together. But it hadn't seemed the right time, after all she'd had her own mother to worry about. I would find the right moment.

Perhaps it was Mum's visit that made me see things slightly differently, but Craig and I seemed to be heading for marriage. At least, that's how I saw it. Not that we talked about it, but we were taking steps together now. For one thing, we were house hunting. The flat belonged to me, and our plan was for Craig to buy a house in his name, then we'd sell both later to buy one house. But, in the middle of our house hunting, Craig changed his mind.

'It's no big deal, Caz, it's just that I'd rather concentrate on my job,' he explained to me after a fruitless expedition to look at a house which I thought had seemed just right.

Craig's concentration on his job meant that it was me who was home most evenings and every weekend now while he was busy. So one weekend Hazel and I left Craig at work and went to stay with our father in Devon. It was late on Saturday night when I said: 'Do you mind if I give Craig a call, Dad?'

'Of course not, Carole, help yourself,' Dad said.

I let the phone ring and ring, but there was no answer.

'That's really strange,' I said, putting the phone down. 'It's late for Craig to be at the golf club.'

'He's probably out with another woman, Carole,' Dad said, laughing. But when he saw the look on my face he added: 'I'm only joking, sweetheart, it was a joke!'

Craig rang the next morning.

'I tried to call you last night, Craig. Where were you?'

'I'm sorry, Caz, but I'd switched the phone off. I was so tired I had an early night.' That wasn't unusual for Craig. It was me who loved talking on the phone, he saw it as an intrusion.

A few days later, back at home, Craig's brother Colin called to see us.

'I'm a golf widow, Colin, did you know?' I said, teasing them both. 'In fact, I think Craig's seeing someone else.'

'Don't be stupid, Caz, of course I'm not,' Craig said. 'When would I find the time?'

'Well, you must be sleeping with someone, it's certainly not me!' I replied. We all laughed. I didn't want an argument but I wanted to get my point across. I realized that we both needed time to adapt to our new situation.

Craig had been in his new job for only a few months yet gradually, particularly in the last month, it had overtaken our lives. He was either at the club or asleep, there was no time for anything else. But there was something wrong, too; there was a distance growing between us and I was beginning to think it wasn't only his job. One night at home, while I was chatting away, he wasn't even bothering to answer.

'What the hell is going on, Craig? When you're here you're not really with me. You might as well be in bloody Finland!' I shouted at him and stomped into the bedroom.

That always did the trick: he'd follow me in, sit on the edge of the bed and we'd talk. But the minutes ticked by and he didn't come. I didn't want to go to sleep on an argument, so I went back out to the living-room. Craig was still sitting exactly where I'd left him.

'You've got to talk to me, Craig, tell me what's going on.'

'I don't know how I feel about anything any more, Carole.' I knew then that this was serious; he rarely used my proper name.

'What do you mean – about me?'

'No, about everything,' he said.

'Craig, are you seeing someone else?'

'Don't be stupid, Carole, I just need some space.' I was crying by now. I needed some answers.

'What have I done?'

'It's not you.'

'What do you mean by "space"? Do you mean you're going away, Craig?'

'I just can't think straight right now.'

'Is it because of the MS?'

'No, of course not. I can't explain it, I feel like I've got a broken heart.'

He started to sob. I climbed onto his lap and, wrapped around each other, we cried and cried. We went to bed, still clinging to each other as though we suspected we would never be this close again.

'I'm going to stay with my brother for a while. I just need some time, Caz, that's all,' Craig said much later as we lay wide awake.

He set the alarm clock and was awake early the next morning. I noticed that he packed very few things, just enough for a couple of days. I was in the bath when he appeared at the bathroom door.

'I'm off now, Caz, I'm going.'

'What's your hurry, Craig, have you got someone waiting for you?'

He quietly closed the bathroom door and I heard the front door bang shut. What a coward! How dare he leave, just like that. I jumped out of the bath, wrapped my bath robe around me, and ran into the kitchen. Opening the kitchen window, I could hear his car engine starting up.

'If you leave like this you're never coming back into my house again,' I shouted across the residents' car park to him, not caring who could see me or hear me.

He came back in but was gone within minutes. I felt complete panic. I knew he'd be back, and I knew that he loved me. But it had been obvious for weeks that he was missing the thought of his summer trip to Finland. And he'd seen me being ill so much of the time recently. Perhaps that was it. Perhaps Craig couldn't cope with me having MS but couldn't bring himself to admit it.

The next day I had an early morning flight to Leipzig. How on earth was I going to get through this? That was all I could think as I drove through empty streets to Heathrow. But again, my job worked its magic. By the time we were in the air and I was busy with passengers I was starting to think that things would sort themselves out. There would be a message on my answer phone when I get home, I thought, as I smiled and served drinks. I even found myself laughing with the crew. But when I arrived home, there was nothing. I changed out of my uniform into the first sweatshirt and jogging pants that came to hand. I went back out to my car, drove to his brother's house and started banging on the door. Eventually it opened.

'Craig, what is going on?' I shouted at him.

'I don't know, Caz, I really don't know how I feel about anything. I've told you that.'

He went inside and I followed, but Craig wasn't intending to have a chat. Instead he made for the kitchen and started to do the washing-up.

'Don't you care at all?' I screamed. 'How dare you do this to me?' I started to hit him, beating his chest like a child having a tantrum. He wrapped his arms around me and I began to sob.

'Craig, tell me honestly. Why are you doing this to me? Don't you love me any more?'

'Of course I do, Cazzy Mac, you know I do. It's not that.'

Five days after Craig had left the flat, I was booked for an overnight trip to Turin. I recognized the dark-haired stewardess with bright red lipstick working in the back half of the plane with me; we'd flown together before and she was so stunning that she wasn't someone you would forget. As we were taking off, strapped in next to each other, Denise Rothwell and I started chatting.

'I haven't seen you for ages, Carole' she said. 'I can't remember when we last flew together, can you?'

'What are you up to these days, Denise?' I asked as I recognized Craig's Glaswegian accent. I didn't want to think about him right now.

'I'm due to qualify as a reflexologist any day,' she said.

'I had that done in Bombay a couple of years ago. I didn't like it, it was really painful. I haven't had it since. Once bitten, twice shy I suppose.'

'Were you unwell at the time, Carole?' she asked quietly.

'Well, I didn't think I was but six months later I was diagnosed with multiple sclerosis,' I said.

'Your reflexologist might even have known and chosen not to tell you.'

'He did tell me I was dehydrated, but that's hardly surprising in the job we do! I know we should drink lots of water, but sometimes I just don't get around to it.'

The 'Fasten Your Seat Belts' sign flashed off and our conversation was cut short as we both made for the galley. The next time we had together was coming in to land in Turin.

'Do you mind me asking how MS affects you, Carole?' she asked as we put on our seat belts for the descent.

It was odd, but I didn't mind at all. She had a calming effect on me and seemed very understanding as I told her about my last relapse. It was the first time I'd ever opened up to anybody about my illness in such detail and to be doing it on a flight struck me as extraordinary.

'Carole, how do you feel about me doing reflexology for you? If it hurts, I'll stop, I promise.'

'Well, I can't lose anything by trying can I? Yes, I'd love that if you don't mind.'

'Have you looked into other treatments for your symptoms yet, like aromatherapy or homeopathy?' she asked.

'Not really. I think of them as luxuries, to be honest. I don't think they could do anything for me.'

'It might be worth exploring them,' she said gently.

Frankly, my head was buzzing with what Craig would do next. I didn't feel I had the time or the energy to explore alternative treatments.

My room in the crew hotel in Turin was huge and very basic. It had enormous windows with wooden shutters but even so it was a gloomy October day and the room was dark. Denise knocked on my door. We'd both changed out of our uniforms and it struck me how glamorous she was, immaculately dressed and not a hair out of place, her trademark bright red lipstick exactly right for her dark colouring. How did she do it, I wondered.

I lay on my bed and Denise put a pillow under my legs. She sat on a chair at my feet and, talking calmly and quietly, she gently began to massage talcum powder into my feet. Then, as she applied pressure with her fingers to different parts of the feet, she explained which organ of the body they were connected to.

'Ouch!' I said as she hit an area which felt uncomfortable.

'Carole, you smoke too much!' she said and laughed. 'It's a disgusting habit!'

'That hurts, too,' I said as she pressed on another spot on my feet.

'You're under a lot of stress, Carole. Have you been poorly in the last few weeks.'

'No, my boyfriend walked out a few days ago. We've been together four years.'

'Ah, that would explain it,' she said quietly, but didn't pry any further.

'Denise, this really is relaxing,' I said a little later.

'I do it for lots of crew,' she said.

We arranged to go to a tiny family-run restaurant that crew used and where I always ordered the same thing – a bowl of pesto, homemade and the best I've ever eaten. There were lots of people at the table, but Denise – who I knew could eat for Scotland and still remain as thin as a rake – and I talked and talked about anything and everything.

'You know, Denise, only a few people at work know about my MS,' I said after I'd been explaining to her how much time I'd had off recently.

'Well, it's no one else's business, is it?' she replied. Instinctively I knew that I could trust her, as though we had an understanding between us. It was marvellous to have someone in the same job listening to me: it was like a weight off my shoulders. But suddenly I felt really tired and said so. Denise smiled.

'So do I. Let's go back to the hotel. You'll get a good night's sleep tonight, Carole,' she said. We walked back to the hotel, our arms linked, and gave each other a big hug. I went to my room and fell asleep, completely relaxed for the first time in months.

'How do you feel this morning then, Carole?' Denise asked as we took off on the flight home.

'I feel brilliant, absolutely wonderful,' I said. 'I slept like a log. I definitely want to have reflexology again.'

She handed me a pile of leaflets about alternative therapies. 'And remember, Carole, if you have one bad experience with a treatment, try someone else.'

'Well, I don't really have the time.'

'Try to make time. Let's keep in touch. And good luck with Craig, I hope it all works out.'

I felt as though I'd known Denise for ages and, although we did contact each other from time to time, my mind was elsewhere. It was to be a whole year before I had reflexology again.

We bumped into each other in the canteen at Heathrow a few weeks later.

'How are your feet, Carole?' Denise said to me, smiling.

'I will have reflexology again, I just don't have the time right now,' I said. 'I know, I have to make the time. Don't tell me,' I said as she smiled and wagged her finger at me, about to tell me off.

Even as I was battling through each day with nothing but Craig on my mind, the idea that there might be alternative ways I could help myself had taken root. Denise was going to change my life, but not just yet.

I kept up the pretence that everything was fine for almost a month. I felt tired all the time and my legs were getting heavier and heavier, but the last thing I wanted was to be sick again. Work had become my escape from an empty flat and a longing for Craig to come home. But I knew something was wrong as I drove to Heathrow airport one bitterly cold November morning. I felt fuzzy, as though I wasn't quite there. Walking up the stairs to the office was a struggle; my legs were like 10-ton weights. I couldn't concentrate on the conversation going on around me, either. It was as though everyone was talking through cotton wool. As I stood at the top of the stairs, my legs gave way. I lost balance and grabbed at the handrail to break my fall.

'Carole, are you all right?' another stewardess rushed over to help me.

'Yes, I'm fine. I just lost my balance.'

I sat on the stairs and after a few minutes eased myself up onto my feet. I felt awful but I wanted to keep some sort of dignity. There was no way I'd be flying today so I set off for the nurse's office.

I just made it inside the door before sinking into the nearest chair, sobbing. I was becoming hysterical and could feel panic rising in me. I had no control over anything. Instead of calmly telling the nurse what had just happened on the stairs, I blurted out everything – Craig, the loneliness, my anger, my illness. She listened until I grew calmer.

'I'll arrange an appointment for you to see the doctor another day,' she said. 'I think you should see Dr Bagshaw.'

'But Dr Mooney is the one who knows me. I trust her.'

'Dr Bagshaw's brilliant, Carole. You'll love him. In the meantime, is there anyone who could take you home?'

The first person I thought of was Craig. I rang him at the golf club.

'Don't be silly, Carole, you know he's off for ten days,' one of the staff said to me when I asked him to fetch Craig to the phone. 'He's gone to stay with his father in Scotland.' I felt stupid.

'Oh, yes, sorry to bother you,' I lied. 'I've rung the club number by mistake. I meant to phone him there. Thanks.'

I drove myself home, feeling sick. Where had he gone? What on earth was going on? There was a message on my answer phone.

'Hi, Caz, just to let you know I'll be away for the next 10 days. I need some time on my own to think.'

I phoned his dad.

'He's not here, Carole. As far as I know he's not coming to stay.'

I phoned his brother.

'Colin, this is making me ill. I've got to know where Craig is.' There was a long silence.

'He's in Canada.'

'He's *where*? What's he doing in Canada?'

'I don't know.'

'He doesn't know anyone there, does he? He's never mentioned Canada to me.' I burst into tears.

There was nothing I could do, and by the end of the week I was back in the Atkinson Morley Hospital for more tests.

'We really do strongly advise you to start a course of steroids, Carole, it's the only thing that will ease the weakness you're feeling all the time.' The neurologist looked at me. He knew my answer, and I went home.

I felt a wreck, and I looked one. I lost half a stone in weight in those 10 days. One evening my friend Liz suggested we should go out to eat. I couldn't swallow anything and later when we stopped off to see her in-laws, they told her they thought I was drunk. I couldn't concentrate, I didn't even have the energy to speak, and I couldn't think of anything to say.

All I could think was that I must make sense of what was going on. I trusted Craig when he said there was no one else. My gut feeling recently had been that there was someone but I'd checked up on him: he had flown to Canada alone. Anyway, he had strict principles; he had lectured friends in the past when they'd had flings. He had always said that if he wanted to sleep with another woman he would split up with me first. There was no way he was having an affair. I knew he would never do that to me.

Then a thought crossed my mind which made everything fall into place. My bet was that he'd had a job offer in Canada and was looking it over before telling me. He knew I would go mad at the thought of him going away again. He probably wanted to make sure it was a job he really wanted before broaching the subject with me. All I could do was wait for him to come home.

I was shocked at how tired and pale Craig looked when I went to see him the day he arrived back in England. He had lost weight, too. He certainly didn't seem like a man who had just had 10 days away from it all.

'How could you disappear like that without telling me, Craig?' I asked him as he sat on the sofa in his brother's living-room.

'I'm jet-lagged, Caz, I can't deal with this right now. Anyway, I left a message on your answer phone. Let's talk tomorrow, eh?'

'No, let's talk now. I've waited 10 days and I want some answers. Who the hell were you with in Canada?'

'OK, I stayed with some people I met at the golf club who have gone out there to live. They said any time I wanted to visit I could, so I took them up on their offer.' His tone was exasperated, as though I was being an inconvenience, a nuisance.

'What were their names?'

He gave me two names. I asked for their phone numbers and he produced them. I knew then that he was telling the truth. He wouldn't give me a number if he was up to anything, would he?

'I've been ill, Craig, I had to go to hospital.'

'Why? What happened? Why didn't you tell my brother?' For the first time since I'd walked through the door, he looked genuinely concerned.

'Why should I, Craig? What difference would that have made?'

But this time I told him everything. I didn't make it easy for him because I wanted him to know exactly what was happening to me. After everything he had put me through why on earth should I protect him any longer from the whole truth about my illness? The days of sparing him the details were gone.

'You know, Craig,' I said when I had finished, 'I wouldn't want you to come back to me out of guilt or because you felt sorry for me. I didn't need your pity, I just needed you. If you were that concerned about me you'd have told me you were going to Canada instead of making me look a complete prat when I rang for you at the golf club. How could you do that to me, you selfish, selfish bastard!'

I went home and slept and slept, for the first time since he'd gone away. I didn't cry and I wasn't angry. I felt confused and exhausted. But when I woke up I felt different, as though something inside me had changed. It was time to stop focusing on Craig. I needed to get back to work. It was the one thing that could get me away from this mess.

7. The Truth Hurts

Rome is one of my favourite cities and, as luck would have it, that's where I was sent that week on an overnight stop. I can sit quite happily at a street café and watch people for hours – and the people-watching in Rome is unbeatable. Or, if I've had enough of the human race on the flight over, I can just look up and lose myself in the magnificent buildings. The only difference this time was that the crew hotel had been changed. Instead of going to an old family estab-lishment on the Spanish Steps we were driven to the new Holiday Inn.

We booked in and arranged to meet for a drink once we'd changed out of our uniforms. We all came down from our rooms one by one into the enormous marble lobby as a woman sat playing the harp. The music sounded strange and other-worldly against the noise of guests arriving and leaving, the ringing of the desk bell and the clatter of luggage being wheeled across the floor by the porters.

While I was waiting for everyone to arrive, I noticed another crew coming in through the front door. I looked at my watch; just coming up to eight o'clock. They must have a really early start in the morning if they're back from having a meal already, I thought. They're probably due for a 4 a.m. alarm call. Then one of them, a man I'd never seen before, walked straight towards me and grabbed my hands.

I pulled away and looked at him. He would pass for an Italian: dark, almost black, hair gelled back from his face and a neatly-groomed moustache. But when he spoke it was with an English accent.

'He's blocking me!' he said, spreading my palms flat and holding them up to show me.

'Do you read palms, then?' I asked calmly. He didn't look like a nutter and anyway I was quite safe. Everyone had gathered around me when they'd heard what this man was saying. I held out my hands to him.

'Yes. He's protecting you. You've lost your grandfather, haven't you?'

Well most people have, haven't they? I thought. But the crew were looking at me now. I didn't know what to say so I laughed and shook my head as we all made for the hotel door.

'Does anyone know who that was?' I asked. I'd like to have known more but it didn't seem the right place to talk.

'That's Graham,' someone said. 'He's a lovely guy, great to work for. He's a cabin service director. I've never seen him do anything like that, though. It was spooky.'

We went for a drink at a tiny bar down a cobbled side street. It wasn't the usual crew haunt, but it had looked so nice from the outside we'd decided to try it out. Then, while we were in the mood for exploring, we braved the rain and made for another bar. When we came out it was pitch dark and, as I stepped onto the slippery cobbles, someone grabbed my arm. I jumped, terrified, but looking round saw that I was face-to-face with the man from the lobby, Graham.

'What are you doing here?' I asked. We were in the middle of Rome; how on earth had he found us?

'I've been standing outside for 20 minutes,' he replied. I could see that the shoulders of his jacket were soaked through. 'I didn't know whether to come in or not.'

'Why? What's the matter?'

'It's your grandad, Carole. I don't want to scare you but he won't let me go to sleep.'

'Come on,' I said, nodding towards the door of the bar. 'Why don't we go in and you can tell me what's going on.' I'd had enough shocks for one evening and I realized how nervous I felt when I found myself ordering a beer. I hardly ever drank these days.

'Right, what do you mean my grandad won't let you sleep?'

'He kept nudging me in bed, Carole. Every time I was about to drop off. In the end, I decided to get up and find you.'

'*Nudging* you?'

'He had boxing gloves on and he kept nudging me in my side. I'm sorry, Carole, does this make any sense to you?'

Graham had my full attention by now. 'My grandad was a boxer,' I said. 'There's no way you could have known that, though.'

'He's certainly stubborn,' Graham said, and I noticed how tired and drawn he looked. He was going to feel dreadful at his early call in the morning, poor thing.

'You're telling me,' I laughed. 'It's a family trait! How did you find me, then? We don't normally come to this bar.' Graham looked sheepish.

'After I got up and dressed, I walked out of the hotel and your grandad was standing on the corner, pointing. By the way, he was in a uniform, Royal Navy, I think.'

'Grandad was in the navy.'

'Every corner I came to, he was there, showing me the way to go. I've followed his directions all the way to you.' It took me a while to think that through.

'Are you psychic, Graham? I mean, what is this all about?' I found myself feeling excited at the thought of this little bit of contact with Grandad, but confused, too. I had certainly never believed in this stuff. But Graham's story was too far- fetched for him to have made it up.

'This has happened to me once before, years ago.' He looked down, not quite catching my eye. 'I'm a bit embarrassed. I don't want to upset you.'

'Don't worry about that, honestly.'

'He wants you to know that everything's going to be all right. But he keeps asking why you are so frightened about having a baby.'

I had never told a living soul about the fear of giving birth that had grown and grown since my diagnosis. They reckon childbirth can trigger a relapse. I'd already had relapses, of course, and I wanted desperately to be a mum. But I had a horror of ending up in a wheelchair. At first it hadn't played on my mind so much but it had become one of those unspoken fears that seemed to be a part of my MS. I couldn't talk about all this to anyone, not even Craig. I certainly couldn't believe I was having a conversation about it with a stranger who claimed to be speaking on behalf of my dead grandfather! I swigged down almost half my bottle of beer.

'I'm not frightened about having a baby,' I said defensively.

'Your grandfather says you're not going to end up in a wheelchair, does that make any sense to you?'

'Not really. He doesn't know I've got multiple sclerosis.'

'Oh yes he does.' There was a long silence.

'Is he still here? Why Rome? Can I contact him now?'

'He'll always be with you, Carole, you can talk to him any time you like in your head and he'll know. He will guide you, if you want him to.'

I didn't know what I wanted. I suddenly felt happy, for the first time in ages, but I'd never believed in this sort of thing. As to Grandad becoming my guide – what did Graham mean? But Grandad was no fool; if ever there was a time I needed some support it was now. He'd made his presence known right on cue.

I wanted somebody else to hear what was going on and looked around the bar. Over at a far table were my captain, the first officer and cabin crew. Graham and I joined them and I told them exactly what Graham had just said. He sat next to me, looking shocked and bewildered. But nobody laughed or disputed it for a minute, even though we all agreed that we didn't believe in it generally. As we were talking it dawned on me that I was speaking openly about MS and even my fears of giving birth. Just a few hours ago I wouldn't have dreamt of doing such a thing. First my meeting with Denise in Turin a few days ago and now this; I was definitely coming out of the MS closet, and I was getting a little help along the way.

I went back to the hotel and climbed into bed smiling. Graham had said I could always talk to Grandad. I didn't know what to say and I felt awkward and shy about talking to thin air. In the end I just spoke inside my head and told him I was glad he'd managed to get a message to me and that I missed him. Speaking to a ghost or a spirit or whatever it was may be the first sign of madness, but all I knew right then was that it was comforting.

Flying home the next day I was trying to decide whether to phone my mother to tell her what had happened. Would it upset her? Would she think I'd gone mad? Would it worry her to think I needed this contact? In the end I thought she should know; it was her father, after all.

'Oh that doesn't surprise me at all,' she said after I'd spent hours agonizing before making the call. 'I often speak to him.'

The things that go on in families without our knowing about them!

'But why do you think he was in Rome, Mum?' I asked. For some reason that had been troubling me since the previous night.

'Well, his mother was a strict Catholic. He'd want to be with her, and Rome is the obvious place for her to be.'

I wouldn't say any of this made much sense to me. Perhaps there are things that are beyond explaining, it was just that the last few years had left me with too many questions buzzing around in my head. Why multiple sclerosis? Why me? Why was Craig in Canada? Why was my life falling apart? The point was that I felt less lonely after Graham claimed that my grandfather was still looking out for me. I decided that, just for once, I would take what had happened at face value. I would stop seeking answers.

Craig came to my flat one evening soon after Rome. I'd been packing his things little by little, and by now everything had gone except one last bin bag. I had even taken all my pictures of him out of the photograph frames dotted around the flat. Hardly a trace of Craig remained. His brother, Colin, was due to pop in later.

'You know, Craig, Colin has been very loyal to you,' I said. 'But he's been a good friend to me in the past few weeks.'

'He was great while I was in Canada, too,' Craig said.

'How could he be? He didn't know where you were.'

'Yes he did, he spoke to me on the phone.'

'But he told me he didn't know where to contact you!'

'Oh well, Caz. He's in a difficult position. I told him not to tell you.'

'How dare *he* lie to me as well. Tell him not to come here.'

'He was just trying to do the right thing.'

'I don't want to see him. And while you're at it, take that last bag of your stuff. If you're going, go properly or you'll find everything sprawled across the lawn.' At last, from nowhere, I was finding some fight.

A few weeks later a parcel arrived from Colin. Inside were heated rollers, a present for helping him get a flight to South Africa to see his mother. There was also a sheet of paper and written on it in black felt tip pen was: 'Dear Carole, Maybe Craig wasn't exactly where you thought. Blood is thicker than water. You'd have done the same if it had been your sister. Love, Colin.' I wanted to speak to Colin, but he was away. I phoned Craig instead.

'I can't believe my brother has done that, I'll be straight over.'

He sat on my sofa and read the letter three or four times. 'I can't believe he would do this to me,' Craig said quietly.

'Are you seeing someone else, Craig?' I asked, thinking that Colin had given me the biggest hint I could ever need. 'If you are, just tell me. If you are lying to me and I find out I shall break every bone in your body.' I shocked myself saying that, but I meant it.

Craig looked me in the eye. 'No, I've told you before. There's nobody else.'

I was dreading Christmas without Craig. What was I going to do? When you've been with someone and they leave, you find that suddenly you have no structure to your life. You're on your own and I had never been alone at Christmas. Then my mum rang.

I began the conversation quite calmly, but I was soon sobbing down the phone.

'Come out here for Christmas, Carole, let me treat you.'

'You can't do that, Mum. It's so much money.'

'Please let me pay for your ticket. I need you to be with me, it's Christmas after all! I don't want you to be on your own.'

'Thanks, Mum. I love you.'

Before I left for Australia, I called Craig.

'I'll be away for two weeks,' I said. 'When I come back you either move back in and we work at it, or you're on your own. I'm not doing this any more.'

The night before I was due to fly he rang and asked to see me. 'I'll be round at eight o'clock, Caz, OK?'

At 10 o'clock I heard his car draw up outside. I listened to his footsteps coming up to my front door and I sat in the silent flat as he rang the bell and waited. If he thought I would let him in when he'd deigned to turn up two hours late, he had another thought coming. Eventually he walked away and drove off. A little while later the phone rang.

'I came round, Caz, but you weren't in. I must have just missed you.'

'You thought wrong then, Craig. I've been here all evening. I was here at eight o'clock, the time we'd arranged. Now, why don't you tell me what's going on?'

Silence.

'If you loved me, Craig, you wouldn't be doing this to me.'

Silence.

'You don't love me any more, do you?'

Silence.

'Tell me you don't love me, Craig,' I screamed.

'I don't love you, Caz.' He spoke so quickly and quietly that I could barely hear him. 'There. That's made you feel good, hasn't it?'

'No, but I needed to know.' I put down the phone. I hadn't believed a word he said. I knew Craig loved me, it was the one thing in life of which I was certain. I couldn't understand what was happening to us.

I really missed Craig in Australia. It was a nice family Christmas, in fact I met my step-sisters, Jade and Zharn, for the first time ever. They lived with their mother in Victoria and we had never been on a visit to Perth at the same time. They were great fun, but all I wanted to do was sleep – not just from exhaustion, but also as an escape. I didn't want to look back and I was too scared to think about the future.

On the flight home, I went through three New Years as the time zones changed and each time the captain announced one I felt a lump in my throat. I didn't know what I was going home to. I lay back in my seat with my eyes closed and turned my situation over and over in my head. I had to face up to my gut feeling. I'd had it for a few months and while I'd been in Australia, thousands of miles away, it had seemed even more clear. Craig was seeing someone else. But in my heart I still felt there was a chance for us; we'd get back together, there would be an explanation for everything, and we would ride this storm.

I arrived at my empty flat on New Year's Day morning, 1994. I had given Craig a deadline. He wasn't at the flat and there were no messages from him, so I had to assume he'd reached his decision. I felt tired and angry. Even now, if I spoke to Craig, he'd ask me how I was feeling. My illness had nothing to do with him any more. It struck me that since he'd come back from Canada I had never wanted him to know about any of my symptoms. I didn't want pity to play any part in his final decision. That would be too demeaning.

I phoned Colin's flat. It was a new year, there was no more time to waste. I wanted to start the year knowing everything, facing up to it, however hard that was going to be. My two weeks in Australia had been an escape but that was over.

'Happy New Year, Colin. So what's going on?' I asked when he came on the phone and told me Craig wasn't there. I couldn't be bothered with wasting any more time.

'Please don't get me involved, Carole,' he said. 'It's not fair. Craig's my brother.'

'I know Craig wasn't where he said he was in Canada, Colin.'

'It's up to him to tell you, Carole. Look, if he hasn't told you by this time tomorrow, then I will. That's the most I can offer you. I'm so sorry he's doing this to you but it's between you and Craig.'

The next morning I rang the golf club. Colin had told me Craig would be at work by 9 a.m. I rang at nine on the dot.

'Happy New Year, Craig.'

'Caz, how was Australia?'

'Cut out the small talk, Craig. If you don't tell me the truth right now about what you were doing in Canada I'll come to the golf club and smash up your car. Then I'll start on you. Is that clear?'

'Look Caz, I'm in the club shop. It's too public. I'll find somewhere more private and call you back. Give me two minutes.'

By the time the phone rang I thought I was going to be sick. Somehow I knew what I was about to hear, but I'd spent four years cherishing Craig for his loyalty and his principles. That was why I felt like throwing up.

'Start talking, Craig. Who were you with in Canada?'

'Maybe I was with someone.'

'Male or female?'

'Female.'

He didn't hang up; he let me scream and shout and swear while he just listened. I couldn't think of words evil or malicious enough to call him but I needed to keep shouting. Then I said: 'I'm coming to the golf club. I'll be there in five minutes.' And I slammed down the phone.

I paced up and down the living-room, up and down, up and down. I was too angry to sit down and too angry to stand still. I had trusted Craig totally and he'd made me feel a fool. I despised him. I didn't know what to do next. What should I do? I had to think clearly.

I couldn't leave it as it was. I needed some answers. I wasn't prepared to wave goodbye to four years without having some reasons. Who was she, for one thing? How long had it been going on? How long had I been a complete fool – days, weeks, months? I wouldn't get anything from Craig so I needed to meet her, his girlfriend. I'd have to shock her into talking to me. But how would I find out who she was?

My sister and I sat in her car in the golf club car park waiting for Craig to finish work. Poor Hazel, once she'd realized how determined I was she hadn't even tried to argue me out of my plan. I was cold and calm and angrier than I'd ever been before. I could guarantee that Craig would go straight to his girlfriend's house after a day of chewing over our phone call. I knew him so well. We would follow and I'd simply take a note of her house and go back the next day.

At last he came through the club door and I sank down in the car seat. He didn't know Hazel's car well enough to take any notice of it; he certainly didn't know her registration number. If anything, he'd be expecting to see my Golf car. She turned her face away as he walked across the car park and climbed into his car.

Hazel shadowed Craig's car as if she'd been doing that sort of thing all her life. I ducked my head below the dashboard so he wouldn't see me and was glad when at last Hazel began to slow down. It had been only a 10-minute journey but every part of my body ached from being curled up, half on and half off the seat.

'I think we're there, Carole,' she said. I lifted my head so that I could just see through the passenger window. We were outside a block of flats. Damn! I hadn't thought of that. Now he'll go in and I won't be able to tell which one she lives in.

'Stay here Hazel, don't follow me whatever happens,' I said and walked round the side of the complex. Craig was walking towards me.

'What are you doing here, Cazzy Mac?' He looked uncomfortable but not as shocked as I'd have expected.

'You didn't think you'd get away with it that easily, did you?' I asked. I was surprised to hear my own voice; I felt like shouting and screaming but I was talking in a normal tone, as if we were discussing which film we'd go to see that evening. 'You're going to tell me exactly what has been going on.'

'I don't know, Caz, honestly. I wasn't unhappy with you, these things just happen, that's all.'

'That's not good enough, Craig. These things don't just happen if you're not unhappy.'

All the time, his new girlfriend was pressing the buzzer on her intercom to open the door. She was probably wondering why it was taking Craig so long to come in. I grabbed the door handle, opened the door and walked in.

'Don't go in there, Caz,' Craig shouted after me as the door banged shut. I was in a huge lobby with a flight of stairs straight in front of me. It was completely silent and for a split second I didn't know what to do. Whoever the girlfriend was, she'd be expecting Craig by now. I looked up and there she was, at the top of the stairs.

'I think you know who I am,' I shouted up at her, my voice echoing around the hard floors and walls of the building.

'You must be Carole.'

'And you are?'

'Tracy,' she said.

I started to walk up the stairs towards her. She looked really scared. 'Don't worry, I'm not going to hurt you,' I said quietly, 'I just need some answers.'

We went into her flat. She wasn't the leggy blonde I'd conjured up in my mind. As we came level with one another I found myself looking down at her. She was short and quite plain, not at all glamorous, but even in my anger I could see that she had an open and honest face. Perhaps a part of me wanted her to be really special. Otherwise, what had driven Craig away from me?

I noticed two glasses of red wine on the coffee table, waiting for Craig to come bounding up the stairs for a cosy evening at home. For a moment I felt a sadness so deep that I was afraid I'd stop being angry. He'd given up all that we'd had for this.

'Tell me what's been going on,' I said, looking straight ahead.

'Where do you want me to start?'

'At the beginning.'

'I met Craig through having golf lessons,' she said, and her Canadian accent suddenly made things fall into place. Craig had travelled out to Canada alone, but only because she was already out there to meet him! The bastard.

'He said you were both really happy together. I asked him out, you see, but he wouldn't go. Nothing happened between us until about a week after he moved out of your flat, Carole, honestly.'

'What about the Saturday night when I rang Craig from my dad's house in Devon?'

'We'd been playing squash that night, that's why he was so late getting home after work,' Tracy said. 'You know, Carole, it hasn't been easy for Craig to leave you, he's been in tears about it all.'

'Don't patronize me!' I got up from the sofa to leave.

'Are there any other questions you need to ask me?' she said. Her niceness irritated me but she had judged the situation well. She seemed to sense just how angry I was and she was making a damn good job of keeping the atmosphere calm. I wanted to hate her but she was making it hard.

'Did you see Craig over Christmas while I was in Australia?' I asked, trying to tie up all the loose ends.

'Yes, I spent New Year at his dad's house in Scotland.'

My God, did that hurt! I felt as though I was going to be sick. It was the first moment that I wanted to kill Craig. He'd taken her to places we'd been together. Everybody in his family knew, except me!

'Thanks for your time, Tracy,' I said as I strode out.

Now, Carole, keep control and hang on to some dignity, I kept telling myself as I walked back down the stairs. But suddenly my legs started to shake and they felt as though they would give way. I had to grip the bannister rail until my knuckles turned white just to stay on my feet. I needed to remain upright and not cry. In my head all I could think was: 'What does he see in her?' I made it to the bottom of the stairs and opened the front door. Craig was still standing where I'd left him.

'You bastard!' I screamed at him. 'You took her to your dad's for New Year and you didn't even have the decency to tell me you were seeing someone else. You are the lowest of the low.' I punched him in the face. He put his hand up over one eye.

'Caz, that really hurt,' he said.

So I punched him again, in the face, then kicked him in the leg.

'I don't know what I'm doing here, Craig, you're not worth it,' I said, calmer now. 'I hope she is.' I nodded my head towards the flat. 'You can be sure of one thing – you'll never get me back.'

I walked away, making for my sister's car, and I could see Hazel's worried face peering through the windscreen. She'd done what I asked, though, and stayed in the car. Craig was shouting after me but I didn't hear a word of what he said. I climbed into the passenger seat.

'Just drive, Hazel,' I said. She started the engine. 'Get me out of here.'

As the car moved off I didn't even look back. I guessed that Craig was watching us disappear, but I had too much pride to check. It was time to leave Tracy, her flat and Craig behind. There was only one question in my mind now. *Why?*

8. Craig's Story

Craig Mitchell was 30 when he left Carole after a four-year relationship to live with Tracy. He was born in Whyalla, Southern Australia, but his family moved back to Glasgow when he was three. He discovered golf in Scotland and is a professional at a club in Surrey. 'I'm not someone who talks too deeply about personal things,' he says, 'but perhaps my experience can help another boyfriend or husband.'

Carole and I are very different types of people. Put her in a room with 10 people and she'll be the centre of attention. She loves that, whereas it doesn't bother me; I'd be the one sitting alone in a corner reading a golf magazine.

I don't come from a family that discusses its feelings very much at all. Carole and her family talk quite openly about how they feel, but I can't do that. It's difficult to get stuff out of me, at least personal stuff. It's just the way I am. I'm not a loner but I'm quite happy getting on with things on my own. There's always a flurry around Carole; her family, friends, colleagues, talking on the phone, visiting. She is a generous person, always ready to help others. That took up a lot of her time when we were together.

When she became ill, her friends were very good. It meant that there were always loads of people worrying about her. I'm always laid back and I can see that could make someone feel neglected. I don't know if Carole feels I neglected her. I think if I had, someone in her crowd would have had a word with me. They're very protective.

The trouble with multiple sclerosis is that most of the time you can't see it. If Carole was out of bed, going to work, being normal, I couldn't see any purpose in making a fuss. I was worried at first, but not too much.

When she rang me from Rio after she was first taken ill I thought it would turn out to be food poisoning or something. Over the next few days the phone calls became more hysterical and I was concerned – but about her, not about what the diagnosis would be. Her dad was worried and he wanted to be the one to go out and be with her, but she wanted me.

She told me she had been drying her hair and because her fingers were numb she couldn't feel her head. OK, so it probably wasn't food poisoning. A virus? Her job involved so much travel she could have picked up anything. But I was more worried by now, we all were.

When I was on the flight to Rio I thought what any bloke would think. Copocabana Beach, blue skies, white sand, naked girls. It wasn't like that at all. It was raining really hard when I arrived and as the taxi driver took me to the hospital we drove past a deserted beach and the skies were grey. In fact, what I remember most are loads and loads of factories.

We reached the hospital and I had no Brazilian money so I couldn't give the driver a tip. I was soaked from head to foot because for some reason he'd insisted on having the windows open. I was taken up to the second floor then down a long corridor. I went into her room and it hit me at last that something was wrong. Things like that aren't real until you see the standard hospital bed and there was Carole. Seeing her in that iron bed was so unfamiliar.

We tried to sleep together in the single bed the first night, but after that I gave up and went on the couch. The thing is, it was all so *boring*; I used to nip out to buy biscuits or cigarettes and have a walk around, anything to relieve the boredom. Carole was having lots of tests but there was nothing for me to do.

Things started to look up when we were allowed to move back to the Rio Sheraton. We had a room with a massive double bed, about 15 floors up. I'm scared of heights but I did try standing out on our balcony one time. I looked down at the hotel's swimming pool and felt as though I was being sucked towards it. And it was still pouring with rain.

I'm not used to hotel life so it was all odd for me. The hotel was fabulous, the food was good, this was really a break. I was still convinced that Carole had a virus and it would clear up; we'd go home and everything would go back to normal. Carole was stressed out, which was understandable. It was a nightmare pushing her wheelchair. She'd keep on: 'Go right, go left, not that way, mind that man, careful!'

Flight crew were always around and there was a crew room in the hotel. I took Carole there several times; she was in her element then, chatting away. She'd been stuck with me for three days in the hospital but the crew gave her a bit of an escape, something else to think about. She was very down in the hospital, but she perked up once we were at the Sheraton.

Every day a posh car arrived at the hotel to take her to the neurologist who had his offices in the town. I went with her for all her tests. In one she had electrodes stuck to her head. 'What do I look like?' she asked. She was laughing; that's very Carole. The neurologist must have made an educated guess about her condition but he wasn't going to say anything, so we came home none the wiser. Copacabana Beach was still empty, the rain lashed down. As a visit to Rio, mine was a washout.

Carole wasn't in a wheelchair when we settled back at home, but she was very weak. She wasn't in bed; she got out of bed every day. It was coming up to the time when I took up my summer job in Finland as a golf pro. The four years I had that job were the best in my working life, there's no doubt about that. It was a complete joy for me to be out there. The rest of the year, in England, I worked lifting boxes in a warehouse. I could only get through those months knowing that Finland was coming up.

When I left, Carole was still having tests and was resting. If she'd needed practical help, perhaps if she'd still been in a wheelchair or couldn't cook for herself, I'd have had a different perspective on things. But she wasn't on her death bed. I didn't have the feeling that I was doing the wrong thing by going away. I didn't have anybody close to me telling me that I should stay, and Carole and I didn't even discuss it. She didn't ask me not to go. I suppose I'm quite a selfish person and I was doing what I loved.

In Finland I had a house on the golf course all to myself. I lived alone out there with lots of space around me, pine forests as far as I could see, all that. In the summer it doesn't get dark there and I felt great all the time. I could give golf lessons all day and all evening if clients wanted them. It was my idea of heaven and, to be honest, once I was out there I forgot all about Carole's situation. I didn't think there was much to mull over at that time. It didn't cross my mind that Carole was going to have an illness for the rest of her life.

I rang her most evenings. One night I called on the phone in the golf club, before I'd finished work, because I knew she was getting her test results and diagnosis. She said: 'I've seen the doctor, I've got multiple sclerosis.' I remember asking her: 'What's that?' It didn't seem like a tragedy to me; she hadn't phoned to say they'd found out what was wrong with her and she had six months to live.

I went back to my house and thought about what she'd told me. It was a bit of a shock. I think everyone's heard of MS but none of us knows what it is. The shock of hearing that long, complicated name and thinking of Carole with it took some getting used to. I suppose it was like that first time I saw her in the hospital bed in Rio; this was something real. It was different in one way, though: in Rio I'd had no idea this would be a condition Carole would have for the rest of her life.

Carole came out to Finland just after she was diagnosed. She was still tired but was on her feet, doing all the normal things. I didn't look at Carole and think: 'This is my girlfriend and she's sick with multiple sclerosis.' It just wasn't like that. MS isn't a limp, it's not visible all the time so it's easy to forget it's there. I never blanked it out of my mind but I simply didn't think about it much.

She had pamphlets on multiple sclerosis and wanted me to read them. I looked at the covers and flicked through them, but I didn't sit down and become engrossed with the subject. I wasn't scared about learning the details but I didn't see the point of reading too much; I tried to explain to her that I would rather cope with each new symptom as and when it affected her. I wanted to deal with it one thing at a time. What was the point in knowing the worst? It might never happen.

It didn't seem important that I never showed an interest in the disease. It all comes back to Carole looking perfectly healthy. As far as I could see she had nothing wrong. Looking back, I should have read everything she gave me. I was too lazy. If I'd been less selfish and more caring at that stage, Carole and I would have had a better chance of being on the same wavelength. It made her angry that I wouldn't read anything.

People like me do things too late; if I had someone close to me who died of MS, *then* I'd go and read about it. As it is, I think more knowledge of the disease might have helped me to help Carole more.

I think on the whole that people thought I was pretty calm and sensible at the time. Some friends would have been quick to put me right if they'd really thought I was handling the situation badly.

Carole and I went to South Africa to visit my mum, Anne Nimmons, who is a nurse. She said to me: 'Do you know exactly what happens to people with MS? Do you know what you're getting into with this?' I thought she was completely missing the point. It didn't make any difference to me, but Mum saw her son having to deal with a girlfriend or perhaps a wife in a wheelchair.

At that stage I needed a third party to talk to – a professional, but a stranger who could sit me down and explain MS and my role as the partner of someone with MS. With a diagnosis like that, everyone focuses on the person who has the illness. That's to be expected. But I needed someone to seek me out and give me information.

It depends on your personality; if our situation had been reversed Carole would have rushed around finding out everything that would have helped me. I feel guilty now because I carried on as though nothing was happening. Carole is a more caring person than I am. Even when she was poorly she was educating herself about MS. She was doing all the work and I wasn't even bothering to read anything.

I know that Carole feels she didn't explain MS enough to me and that she hid some of her symptoms. But it's not fair that she should take any responsibility at all. She has the illness and, being Carole, would have wanted to communicate. Our lack of communication was my fault.

If I think back I really can't remember many relapses or bad days. She'd get tired – but we all do. We once had to leave a party early when she felt unwell, but things like that are no big deal. I know her legs would get wobbly or she'd have pains in her eyes, but I never thought that everything boiled down to multiple sclerosis. Her job put her under a lot of pressure, too, and goodness knows what so much flying does to your body.

Apart from that first bout of MS when I flew out to Rio and Carole was in a wheelchair, her MS didn't show. At least, it didn't show to me. So it never made her less attractive to me – either physically or mentally. We hadn't considered children as a definite plan so I never thought about the effect having a child would have on her. It may put stress on a woman with MS, but I don't know anything about that. Carole wanted children, she has always loved babies, but I didn't at that time. I wasn't thinking along those lines.

Someone left me years ago and I spent a long time wondering why she'd gone. You can waste years trying to find an explanation, but there isn't always one reason. If Carole had suffered a really bad relapse perhaps people could have looked at us and thought: 'Oh well, she's in a wheelchair and he can't cope.' But the illness wasn't everything. It wasn't the thought that I couldn't cope with Carole having MS that made me leave her, definitely not.

We were a very close couple but I didn't feel I *had* to stay with Carole because she was ill. I wasn't walking around feeling unhappy for months, I just happened to meet someone else. It was a bit of a shock, to be honest. But I wouldn't do things differently if I had my time again. It's just that we drifted apart for no specific reason.

The big thing that changed in my life at that time was that I no longer had my six-month job in Finland to look forward to. One thing fed off the other for me: I enjoyed my time in England with Carole because I knew I had Finland coming up. She used to come out to visit me and it was really exciting. Driving to the airport to pick her up was like meeting for the first time all over again. I loved all that.

My work in Finland made my boring warehouse job in England bearable. The fact that there was always change going on was important to me.

When you're living with somebody every day you don't realize a gap is growing between you or that the other person is changing. It's gradual. When I met Carole she was happy-go-lucky and loved her job. She changed over a period of time, but not only because of her illness. She'd had several family and friends' deaths to deal with and being off work made her go into debt. These things are bound to change someone, and their attitude towards life. These are all things which could have contributed to me meeting someone else and ending the relationship.

If I'd been the one with MS then Carole would have made me breakfast in bed, taken me to the doctor's. I never once tried to put myself in her shoes, which might have been a more sympathetic thing to do. Carole would be shouting and screaming at me in frustration, but it all flew over my head. I'm not the type to get like that, I just can't be bothered.

I found after I'd left Carole that if the subject of MS came up in conversation sometimes I'd chip in, sometimes I wouldn't. I'm no expert on it.

Of course, the longer time goes on the greater the chance that she will have a relapse. But while we were together I didn't think about her dying, or me needing to look after her when she was as good as dead. That's not how it works. I think now we'll be friends.

I sometimes have an image of someone in a wheelchair with a rug over her knees, dribbling. It will be difficult if Carole has a relapse; she's very independent and it will hit hard. Carole would be a good person to have around if I was ill. It seems there's no justice in this world.

9. A Time to Heal

The daytime was easier once I arrived in Australia. I could sit by my auntie's pool or climb in to Mum's car and go to the beach. As I lay with my eyes shut and felt the sun's scorching heat flood through me, my mind emptied.

But at night every time I closed my eyes all I saw was Craig or, even worse, Craig with Tracy. It was a nightmare. I had come to the other side of the world to get them out of my life. Since I'd arrived in Perth to stay with my mum I had learned that all the time I was thinking about Craig I would never get any rest. Then one night I'd fallen straight to sleep only to wake up with a start at 2 a.m., crying over a dream in which Craig and I were still together, still a couple, but he was leaving me.

I was beginning to see some things more clearly. I had learned to get up rather than lie wide awake in the dark. I'd quietly move around my room with its double bed and mosquito nets draping the windows. I would take some paper from a drawer and write page after page, trying to put into words all my anger and disbelief in letters addressed to Craig that I knew I would never send. Why, Craig? Was she worth it? How could you do this to me?

The questions crowded my mind almost to daybreak, then I'd have a few hours' sleep before Mum woke me up and I began another day. I'd left cold, grey, damp London just a few days before. Here the grass in Mum's garden was so dry that it crunched under foot and the birds flying from tree to tree were still a shock – parrots, budgerigars, cockatoos. It was foreign and exotic and it suited my mood, a break with the past and a new future. It was just that I couldn't even begin to imagine what that future would be. I had lost my best friend because he had betrayed me. Yet I needed to talk to him. I had to keep reminding myself that Craig wasn't my friend any more and I missed that most of all.

All the time I was waiting for a relapse with a fear that bordered on panic. Surely, if it's stress that triggers them, I'll get one now, I thought. The worry was like a mantra, humming inside my head. I wasn't well at all; my head felt heavy and I was dragging my body around like a ton weight. I was weepy and miserable and it was an effort talking to Mum and her husband, Ivan, when they came home from work – not because they weren't interested, but because I didn't feel that I should burden them with my problems to worry about. It all made my head spin.

I was doing exactly as the doctor had ordered, though. I could feel hot tears behind my eyes as I thought of British Airways' Dr Bagshaw and his blackboard.

'This, Carole, is you,' he'd said in his office at Heathrow airport as he drew a cup on the blackboard while I sat crying. Why, I had asked, had I coped with everything over the past few years but been floored by my boyfriend leaving me?

'Now remember, everyone has different coping mechanisms. This is your grandad's death.' He drew a shape inside the cup. 'These are other family deaths, here's your MS, and this is Craig.' He started to draw long lines spilling over the top of the cup.

'Your body can't cope with this one last thing right now. It will in time, but it will be like a wound. You should expect it to mend slowly, then hurt a little when it gets knocked, then mend more until finally the hurt goes away. You'll be left with a scar, but you will be healed. So you won't ever be quite the same again, but neither will you be hurt like you are now.' He turned away from the blackboard rubbing the chalk from his fingertips.

'If I could give you one thing that you feel would help you, Carole, what would you want?'

I had looked at Mike Bagshaw, dapper in his tweed jacket and bow tie, and answered without really thinking. 'I want my mum.' It hit me that what I needed was to be looked after. I simply needed a hug.

'Then I'm signing you off for three months and I suggest you get yourself on a flight to Perth as soon as you can. Go home, you're really not fit for work. You're not flying today.' He handed me another tissue from the box he'd put by my side on his desk and looked at me kindly. 'Good luck, and I'll see you when you come back to work.'

So here I was, just a month after my Christmas visit. I hadn't given Mum much warning that I was coming so she couldn't take time off from her job as a book- keeper. The first morning, left alone in the house, I had walked out through the patio doors and the heat hit me like a sledgehammer. It was 42°C and rising. There was no way I could move around in that so I retreated into the cool of the house for the rest of the morning, nursing my jet lag. I munched through huge wedges of water melon feeling dazzled by the brightness of the sun, the deep blue of the sky.

Mum came in through the front door at lunchtime and put her arms around me. 'I can't believe I've got you all to myself. Give me a cuddle!'

I knew I had made the right decision to come to Perth to heal. At the airport the previous day Mum had rushed out from the crowd waiting for my flight, stooped down under the barrier and hurtled towards me as I stood with my elbows resting on the luggage trolley, my head in my hands. I'd kept complete self-control until the moment I'd seen her, then I had felt a wave of relief. At last I could cry, and it would be easier to cry with my mum there to hold me.

Now here I was preparing lunch in her spotless kitchen, its huge windows looking out on to the patio.

'I've made us a sandwich, Mum,' I said. As I hugged her, I felt a lump in my throat because I knew I'd have her around for months this time rather than just days.

We sat on the wicker chairs in the dining room, a ceiling fan above us making a quiet whooshing noise as it turned slowly.

'I think I'll join a gym, I need to get fit and healthy,' I said with more conviction than I really felt. 'It'll give me something to do while you're at work.'

'I know, why don't you drive me back to work in the afternoons then you can have my car and go exploring? It's better than sitting here brooding.'

So my gentle routine began. I found a gym where the instructor, after a chat about my illness, gave me a sheet of very mild exercises and showed me how to use weights. I couldn't do much, nor for long, but it was a first step.

Mum's car gave me the freedom to go to the beach or make the 20-minute journey from her house in Leeming across to my Auntie Angela's bungalow so I could use her pool. As I grew used to the heat I added a little sunbathing to my schedule. But I couldn't escape the nights.

I wonder how many never-to-be-posted letters I wrote to Craig during those early days? I had not had a chance – correction, he had never given me a chance – to tell him what I really thought or felt about the way he had treated me, and this was my way of dealing with it. I found a shoe box and at the end of each flurry of writing I would put the new pages in on top of the old. They all said the same thing but it was beginning to feel good being angry at Craig. It seemed to put me back in control. I needed my thoughts to be given an airing. I was me now, not me and Craig. But all the time that old familiar tingling was creeping up my legs and along my arms as the tiredness turned into exhaustion.

On my fifth day in Perth panic set in. All day, like a little girl, I had wanted my mum. I wanted to talk to her alone, I wanted her full attention. But I couldn't have her to myself. First she had to go to work. Then, at lunchtime, she told me that she and Ivan had friends coming round for drinks that evening.

'Oh, that'll be lovely,' I lied.

That afternoon I lay on the beach alone, thinking hard about my new situation. I was single, I had MS, what man was ever going to look at me again? And if they did, when would I tell them I'd got MS? And if I told them, how would they react? What if I met someone I really liked and then they ran away? I felt panic as my situation became painfully clear to me. I could hate every man I met for the rest of my life, that would be one way of protecting myself. Or I'd have to do something about this sense of panic. I couldn't keep all this inside me; I thought my head would burst. I needed to talk to Mum.

I thought Mum's friends would never leave that evening. I was very poor company as they drifted from the living-room out on to the patio, talking and laughing. I couldn't think of anything to say to them but I was scared that if I didn't open up to my mum now, I never would. I realized that I hadn't spoken to anyone properly about my MS, and once Craig had gone I'd brought down the shutters. At last the guests started to leave, and mum and I heard the car doors banging and Ivan having a joke with one of his friends as we sat down at the table on the patio. We looked at each other.

'I can see the hurt in your eyes, darling,' Mum said to me, and I burst into tears. She dragged her chair next to mine and put her arms round me while I sobbed and sobbed. Ivan wandered through the patio doors and, realising what was going on, went back into the house quietly.

'It hurts so much, Mum. It hurts so much.'

'I know, darling, I know,' she said; there were tears in her eyes.

'How could he have done that to me?'

'Carole, someone wonderful will come along. I know it.'

'Oh yes, I'm sure. Who'll want me now?'

'What do you mean, darling?'

'I've got MS, Mum. Multiple sclerosis. No man will want me now!'

'But you're still *you*, darling. That hasn't changed. The right man will love you for who you are, with or without MS. It's just that the right man hasn't come along yet. The two things haven't got anything to do with one another. You must believe that.'

'I've wanted to talk to you all day, Mum, but I couldn't get you alone.'

'Oh darling, why didn't you tell me? I'd have told everyone to go away if I'd known.' I began to cry again.

'I haven't been able to cry about being ill before, Mum, I've never had anyone to cry with. I have to keep putting on a brave face and I was doing really well until Craig ...' She put her arms around me again.

'You know, Carole, I felt that if we didn't mention MS it might go away. But it doesn't, does it?'

'It's easy to lie about it, Mum, because a lot of the time you can't see it. That's what I do. I hid the symptoms from Craig because he didn't show much interest. And anyway, he didn't understand what I was going through. I've hidden them from you because I didn't want to upset you. You were a long way away. I didn't think you needed to know all the details.'

Mum put her hand over mine and gave it a big squeeze. Still holding tight, she looked at me.

'It's the hardest thing when your child is ill, darling. Any mother will say the same thing. I want to make you better and I feel helpless. I'd have done anything to prevent this happening to you. I'm only just coming round to accepting that you are ill. All I could feel at first was panic that there was nothing I could do to stop it.'

'Oh Mum, look at us. We've both been trying so hard to protect each other we've never given ourselves the chance to say how we really feel.'

'Well, I know now that not talking about it doesn't make it go away!'

'That's the trouble, nothing will make it go away.' The tears started to roll down both my cheeks and Mum wiped them away with her fingers.

'No, but we can make sure we don't give in. We've got to get your fight back, darling. We'll do this together. I'm here for you and I'll do anything I can to help you learn to live with your illness. I just want you to be happy. You deserve that.'

'Yes, but look what happened with Craig. He's gone off with someone else and I thought we were made for each other. Who is ever going to want me again? How would I find the right time to tell them I've got MS? What do I say to them? That's all I kept thinking at the beach this afternoon. Oh, God. What am I supposed to do?'

'Don't get things muddled up, darling. Having MS doesn't mean you'll never be happy again. That's up to you, you will have to make that happen. You've got as much love and support from me as you want.'

'I know, Mum. But I don't know where to begin.'

'You've gone through two traumatic events, Carole. You've been diagnosed with MS and you've lost the man you love. But you've lived! You've got through both and it's time to start rebuilding your life, think positive things, look ahead.'

'You're right Mum. I don't want it to get the better of me but I think it has lately. I've lost all my strength. I feel so weak.'

'You'll get your strength back, darling. You'll be fine.'

We stood up and she gave me a big hug.

'*Que sera, sera*, darling, What will be, will be. I love you so much. Don't worry. We're going to work at this together.'

We linked arms and went back into the house. I felt tired, exhausted in fact, but I had a feeling that things were going to look different from now on. At least I had one ally, and talking so openly about being ill made me feel differently about it, made it seem less frightening and more manageable. I went to bed and fell into a deep sleep.

The next morning I woke up thinking about Craig, with that ache of wanting my best friend with me. I knew Mum was right, I would meet someone else, but how much time would it would take to learn to live without Craig? I had a lot to think about and the best place for that was by my auntie's pool. I could lie there for as long as I wanted.

I drove the 20 minutes or so to her bungalow at Armadale in the hills and made myself at home. Sun cream, sunglasses, sun lounger, and a book I wouldn't read. I slipped a Diana Ross tape into my Sony Walkman, put the ear plugs in and lay down. The track 'Reflections' came on and the words made me shiver. I couldn't seem to escape my memories, they were in everything I did these days. I looked up at a sweeping curve of palm fronds and their sharp edges blurred as I remembered my flight out to Perth. I really had thought my life was coming to an end. The tears started and I rummaged blindly in my bag for a tissue.

I spent days and days by that pool or alone at the beach and it gradually dawned on me that I was desperate for change. I wasn't happy with a lot of my memories. I needed a new beginning and I wanted to find my own identity. Living with Mum and Ivan made me notice something I'd been missing for ages: the freedom to be myself. With them I could cry, throw a tantrum, shout or laugh. Craig used to look at me as though I'd gone mad if I showed my frustrations. Then I'd end up driving round and round south London until I had calmed down enough to go home to him.

I soon realized that coming to Australia was the best decision I could have made. I was beginning to sleep more and feel a little better when I woke up. I slowly tried to convince myself that I *could* feel well. I might have MS but I hadn't been given six months to live; my task was to adapt, learn my limits and get to know my strengths. Then I could get on with living.

Ivan looked more relaxed, too. The poor man, so big-hearted and kind, must have been stunned when I turned up in such a sorry state. But now he could see I was making some progress and felt I was ready for some joshing when he came home from working at the drilling company he owns.

'Hello, stepdaughter, and how are we feeling today?' His blue eyes sparkled and a huge grin cut through his beard.

'I'm extremely well, thank you, stepfather.'

It became our ritual, every evening, as the two of us slowly got to know one another on this visit, my longest with Mum since she had married him. His sense of humour was just what I needed as I began to recuperate. I would chat to him as he lavished care on his collection of Ducati motorbikes and soon slotted into his easy-going way of life.

One afternoon I found myself pacing up and down the drive of Mum's house, waiting for Ivan as he'd borrowed her car. I was due at a friend's house to babysit in three minutes and he had promised he would be here. At last Ivan came down the road looking far too big for Mum's little old banger.

'Where have you been?' I screamed. 'I've been tearing my hair out.'

'Well, I'm here now, kiddo. Don't worry.'

I climbed into the car and started the engine. Oh great, no petrol.

'Ivan, there's no petrol in it! I'm going to be late.'

'Never mind, kiddo. Take the Saab.' He threw me the keys to his brand new car – typical Ivan, he'd have done the same if it had been a Ferrari. Material things don't mean much to him. I got into the driver's seat and drove off in seventh heaven. Then the problems began. I decided to put on some music; Mum's Elvis CDs were neatly piled in one side of the glove compartment, Ivan's Jethro Tull in the other. While I was getting into a muddle over them, the car phone rang. Oh no, how do I use it? It kept ringing, on and on. It might be urgent. Just as I discovered how to answer it, the traffic lights ahead turned red. Thank goodness!

'Hello darling, how are you getting on with the car?'

'Fine, thanks Mum. It's a dream.' It was a white lie but a few miles further down the road and I felt as though I'd been driving Ivan's car all my life.

Ivan influenced my diet, too. It was easy to eat healthily in Perth, with fresh fruit and salads all I wanted in the hot, hot weather. Ivan took Mum and me to their favourite fish restaurant so that I could discover oysters and garlic crayfish, and he was a great barbecue cook, too. I didn't need to lift a finger but was enjoying the perfect diet, with lots of treats thrown in!

I started to look at my symptoms in a different way. I'd been waiting for the relapse and it hadn't come. But I still had a tingling in my legs and arms and I stopped pretending that I hadn't. If I felt tired, I rested. It was really a question of putting the focus on me, instead of always worrying about what other people would think. I didn't know how I would cope with that when I was at work, I couldn't just keep taking days off.

After a few weeks I started to feel fantastic, and I looked much better. I'd lost a stone in weight before I arrived in Perth, but it had been an unhealthy weight loss from being too angry and upset to eat. Now, with my trips to the gym every other day and a good diet, my body was beginning to tone up. The tan helped, too.

'I'm so proud of you, darling,' my mum said to me one day, 'you look well and happy again.'

'Well, there's nothing like a bit of motherly love to help along the way!' I said, and gave her a hug. I doubt whether she'll ever know what a relief it was to me that she was there to talk when I needed her.

'I'm beginning to be able to tell when you're not feeling too good, Carole,' she said.

'How?'

'You move just a bit slower and you have a look, a sort of tiredness. There's no sparkle in your eyes.'

'I didn't realize it showed.'

'You don't talk as much, either!'

'Well, at least that's a blessing in disguise.' We laughed, but I thought back to all those times I'd come home from work and pretended to Craig. I hadn't talked to him then because I didn't think he was interested. But he must have noticed I wasn't well. Now that I'd come clean with Mum, the lack of communication between Craig and me made me feel sad and angry. I felt bitter, too.

One day I went to Cottesloe Beach with Katie MacDonald, an English girl I had got to know. We always had the beach to ourselves; Australians are too sensible to sunbathe. We had our usual cappuccino and apple cake at the beach café then settled on the soft white sand.

'Would you take Craig back if he asked?' Katie asked out of the blue.

I didn't answer straight away but sat staring at the sea, scooping the sand through my fingers. It hit me just how much I was missing him.

'Yes, today I think I would.'

I looked along the beach, as though imagining him walking towards me, and I felt so angry with myself. How could I be so pathetic?

That evening, after dinner, I told Mum what had happened.

'Mum, I can't believe I could think like that.'

'Is that what you really want, to have him back?'

'No! He doesn't deserve me. It shocked me when I said I would.'

'You know I'll stick by you whatever you decide.'

'Honestly Mum, I'll never take him back. I can't.' I burst into tears. 'He lied to me. Why didn't he just tell me the truth? I deserved the truth. I'll never forgive him for making me look such a fool!' I threw yet another tissue into the swing bin and looked at Mum.

'I'll go to bed now, Mum. I'm tired.'

She gave me a big hug. 'Good night, darling.'

I sat on my bed, shaken by how angry I felt, and thought about the days before I'd flown out. I had met Craig in a pub to discuss our bills. I hadn't told him I was going to Australia, just that I would be away for a while. It was the first time since we'd met each other that I'd planned something this big without him knowing about it, and it felt odd. But he had seemed like a complete stranger and I had looked at him across the table, despising him. The man I'd fallen in love with four years before just didn't exist any longer. This man was a coward. I couldn't even remember what we had said to each other, but it didn't amount to much.

It wasn't Craig I missed, it was *someone*. There's a big difference between being single from choice or single because you've been dumped. Before I'd been getting on with life secure in that feeling of being part of a couple. But it had all been a big lie. I hadn't chosen to leave Craig, he had chosen to leave me. I hadn't been ready to be single.

I couldn't imagine being with anyone else, though. I couldn't conjure up a picture of me with another man, any man. I hated men. That was so obvious I could have had it tattooed across my forehead. Nobody was ever going to hurt me again the way Craig had, the barriers had gone up. I might be looking a bit better but I certainly wasn't ready in my mind for a new relationship. If any man had asked me out in Perth I don't think I'd have given him the time of day! Meeting someone was the last thing on my mind.

I thought it would be difficult for me to be a guest at a wedding just then but watching my auntie get married again was a turning point of my stay in Perth. It was a baking hot day and as I stood by her swimming pool to witness her taking her vows I had to bite my lip to stop the tears coming. Angela had been through so much in the last two years; first her husband had died, then her son, then her father. But today she looked at peace as she and her new husband stood under an arbour of lace and pink roses for the photographer.

'How are you feeling, darling?' Mum came over to join me while the other guests wandered around the garden.

'It's funny, Mum, I feel really happy. I'm pleased for Angela and I was just thinking that she has been through hell and survived, so perhaps there's hope for me yet!'

Now that I was feeling stronger I began to worry about a problem which I'd pushed to the back of my mind. Before I'd left London I had arranged with my closest friend, Julie, that we would share a house when I went home. Tenants had already moved in to my flat, thank goodness. I didn't want to go near there for a while, with all its memories. I'd been anxious that Julie wouldn't be able to find anywhere and I would go back to London homeless. Then she rang.

'Carole, I've found a terraced house in Wimbledon. What do you think?'

'Do you like it?'

'Yes, I really do. It's small but it's lovely. I think it's just right for us.'

'OK, let's go for it.'

I signed the letting contract by fax and Julie, whom I'd known since I was 17 when we were both nannies, moved in while I was still in Perth. It was a weight off my shoulders. Now I knew that when I landed at Heathrow I would have a home to go to and a good friend to share it with.

Over the weeks the tingling in my arms and legs had eased away; I hadn't even noticed until I realized that I had not felt ill for a long time. As my visit went into the third month I was joined by a cousin and her friend on holiday from England. I found I had the energy to enjoy going out for meals, shopping trips and exploring. We went walking in the bush and even go-karting. I was glowing with health. I wouldn't quite say I was slim, but it's amazing what a tan can do for you. I felt focused, too. I wanted to take care of myself and I wanted to feel this well all the time.

Part of me had begun to accept what had happened with Craig; people do meet other people. I still felt he had handled the situation badly and had made me look an idiot, but I didn't feel so angry. I could even see that it hadn't been easy for him, either. When he'd first met me I didn't have a care in the world. Look how much had happened to me since then! He certainly hadn't understood what I'd been going through since I had been diagnosed with MS, but then neither had I. I'd had months to think things through in Australia with no distractions. I'd realized I had to take some of the blame.

I recalled what my doctor had said to me before I had come to Perth – that Craig walking out on me had hit the hardest because I was left alone to cope with it. He had been with me through everything that had happened before. I didn't want him with me through anything else, though. I knew I didn't want Craig back. The truth was, I seemed better off without him.

It was on my birthday, 6 April 1994, that it hit me that my visit was coming to an end. I had one more week left. Then it was just four days. Time was racing. I woke up on the day I had to fly back to London with a sick feeling in the pit of my stomach. I wanted the day to be over with. Mum and I spent breakfast avoiding eye contact.

'Shall we go out for coffee and do some shopping, darling?' she asked, looking so sad.

'That's a really good idea. There's no point in moping around here.'

While we were out I gave Mum the slip and bought her a card saying how much I loved her. I knew I'd never be able to say it without floods of tears – from both of us. We went home and I put the card under her duvet while she was in the bathroom. I packed the last few bits and pieces. Should I tear up all those angry letters I'd written to Craig in the middle of the night or take them home? I squeezed them into a suitcase. I was drying my hair when Mum caught my eye as she passed the door to my room. We both burst into tears and clung to each other. We stood holding each other for ages before either of us could speak.

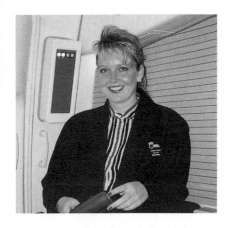

New girl: Carole is flying at last, a dream fulfilled as she becomes a stewardess with British Airways in 1988.

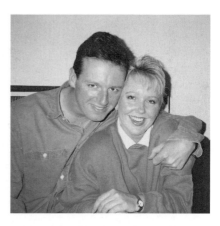

Golf-mad boyfriend Craig Mitchell admits now that he could have been 'more caring'.

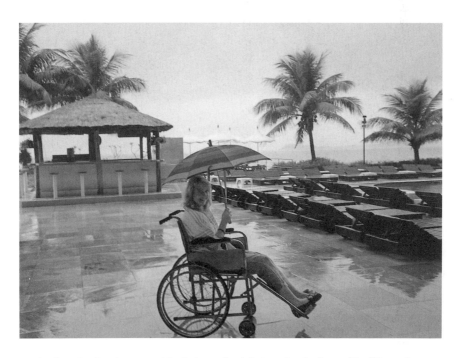

Rio in the rain: Carole was suddenly in a wheelchair and nobody could tell her what was wrong. It would be three months before she knew she had MS.

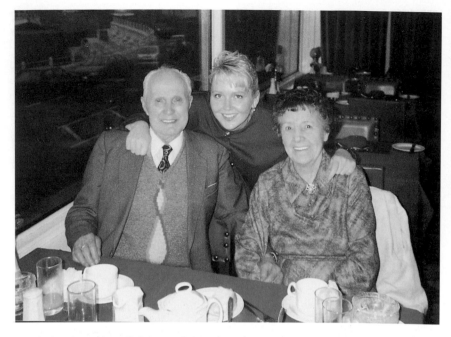

Family bond: Carole with her grandparents, Peter and Annie, at a New Year dinner in Banff, Scotland, in 1992. Three months later her grandfather died.

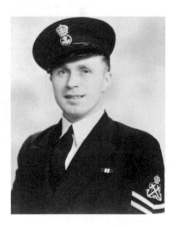

Carole's maternal grandfather, Peter Crawford, as a handsome young man in his navy uniform (see page 90).

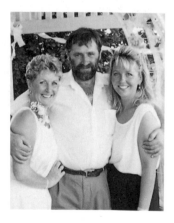

Carole with her mother and stepfather, Ivan, at her aunt's wedding in Perth, Australia, in 1994.

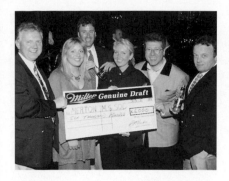

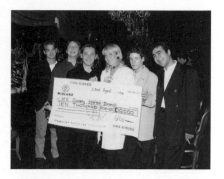

First charity event, 1995: Carole with her father *(left)*, DJ Neil Fox and others, with a cheque for £6,000 raised for MS research. *Reproduced by kind permission of Jon Bushell.*

Second charity event, 1996: £10,000 raised this time and Carole celebrates with members of the cast of the TV soap 'EastEnders'. *Reproduced by kind permission of Jon Bushell.*

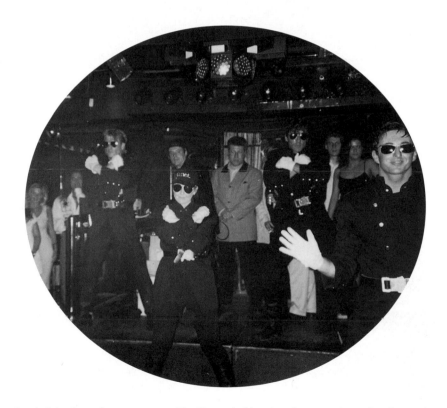

Carole joined a male revue group, The Untouchables, in a dance routine at her first charity event. 'Shock people into knowing that people with MS can do anything,' they said.

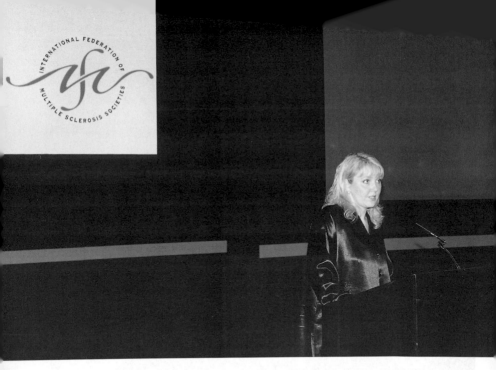

Stage nerves: Carole addresses the International Federation of MS Societies at the Science Museum, London. *Reproduced by kind permission of Uppa Commercial Photographers.*

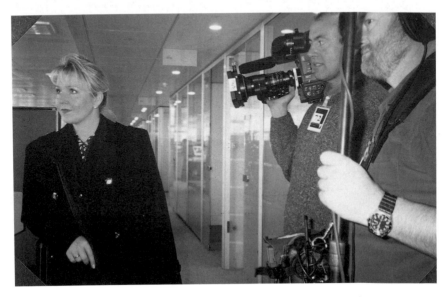

Star quality: Carole at Heathrow Airport in 1995 during the making of the television documentary *The Pulse*. Filming had to be postponed after she was taken ill.

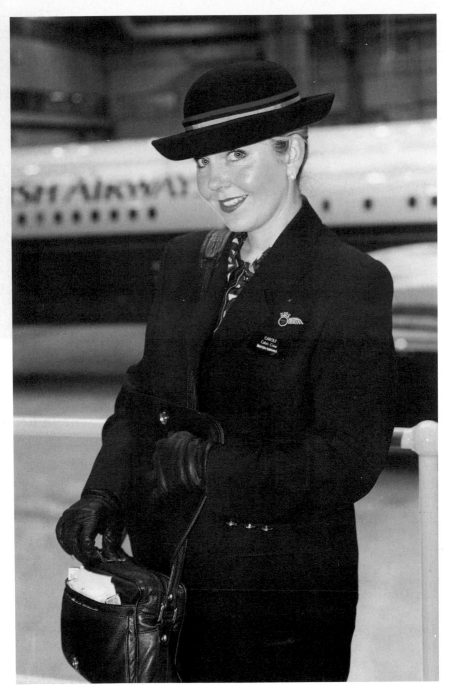

New look: Carole at the end of filming, well again and looking smart in the new British Airways uniform. *Reproduced by kind permission of Express Newspapers.*

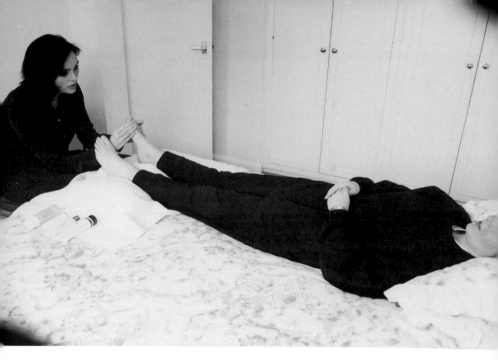

Self-help: Carole has reflexology from her friend and fellow-stewardess, Denise Rothwell. Denise was killed in a car crash a few months later. *Reproduced by kind permission of Express Newspapers.*

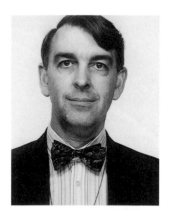

Dr Mike Bagshaw, head of British Airways' medical services. 'He has always trusted me to be honest with him,' Carole says.

MS victim Carole plans nightclub fundraiser

● British Airways stewardess Carole Mackie

by SHAILJA CHIBBER

BRITISH AIRWAYS stewardess Carole Mackie is planning a big night out to raise funds to help fight a crippling disease of which she is a victim.

Multiple sclerosis sufferer Carole (28) is taking over the top West End nightclub Stringfellows on May 23.

She is hosting a 'Wild Night Out' for the Multiple Sclerosis Society.

She is inviting friends, colleagues and supporters to join the fun while helping fund research into the illness which struck her four years ago.

Now a short-haul stewardess, Carole was diagnosed as having multiple sclerosis

after a work trip to Rio de Janeiro.

Her fingers and chest had become completely numb overnight.

The disease hits the central nervous system, stopping messages being sent properly to other parts of the body.

In Carole's case, it follows a pattern of relapse and remission. For long periods, she feels fine, then she hits a bad patch.

Anniversary

But she is optimistically battling on and hopes to raise awareness about the disease as well as funds for research.

The event also marks the tenth anniversary of her local branch of the MS society in Merton.

She said: "I am indebted to

the organisation and hope to raise £10,000 from the event for both research and MS awareness."

The Wild Night Out will feature Capital Radio DJ Neil Fox and the all-male revue The Untouchables.

Celebrity guests will draw the bumper raffle. The first prize is two BA Club class tickets to a destination of the winner's choice. Other prizes include a session behind the controls of a jumbo jet simulator, a weekend holiday break and a year's free membership of Stringfellows.

Tickets, at £10, are available from BA special services at Heathrow's T1 and T4 and the crew shop at both Heathrow and Gatwick. Donations can also be made at these points.

Posthouse airport hotels net £4,500 for charity

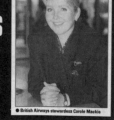

● The Forte Posthouse hotels at Heathrow and Gatwick have raised more than £4,500 for Scope - formerly the Spastics Society.

The money was raised by staff and guests in a range of fundraising events. Funds from Heathrow's Posthouse totalled £1,350, with the Gatwick Posthouse raising £2,168.

The year-long Forte Posthouse Family Challenge was originally expected to raise £81,000, but money has risen to a staggering £143,096.

Carole's first appearance in a newspaper made her livid at the use of the word 'victim'. 'I realized people needed to be educated,' she says.

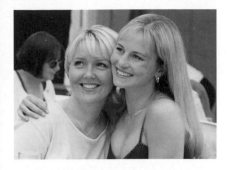
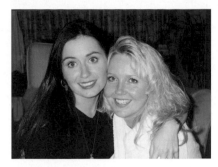

Friends: Carole with former flatmate Anna *(left)* and friend Maxine *(right)*.

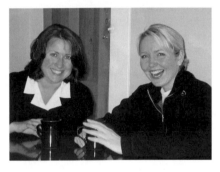
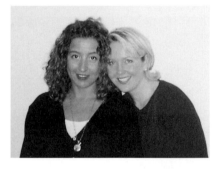

A friend in deed: Carole with Julie, who organized a house for them to share while Carole was recovering in Australia.

Helping hand: Carole with her friend Sara, who has guided her through a programme of aromatherapy and massage.

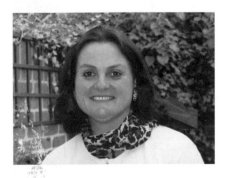
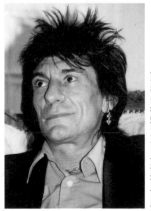

Carole's manager at BA, Maggie Sheppard 'My wish for Carole is that she has one long remission.'

Rolling Stone Ronnie Wood *(right)* wrote the Foreword in memory of his great friend, Ronnie Lane, who died in 1997.

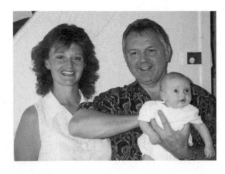

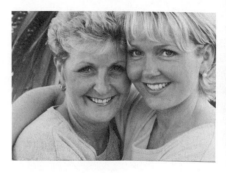

Carole's dad, Ron Mackie, with his wife Helena and little daughter, Abi.

Carole with her mother, Isabell, in Perth, Australia at New Year 1997.

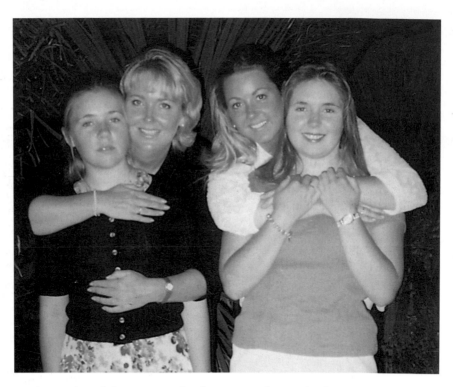

Family: Carole with her sister Hazel and stepsisters Zharn and Jade in Perth, Australia.

'I don't want you to go, my darling. What shall I do without you?'

'What shall *I* do without *you*?'

'Come on, Mum, let's enjoy our last day together.' We laughed and went to find some tissues. We both knew we shouldn't waste the whole of this precious day crying.

It was a different story at the airport. We all stood outside the building as I wanted a cigarette but eventually the dreaded words came drifting over the tannoy. 'British Airways, Singapore–London flight is now boarding. Please proceed ...' Everybody was there; Ivan and Mum, my cousins, friends, all crying. I picked up my hand luggage and set off ahead of them but I had only gone a few yards when I dropped my bags.

'I don't want to leave you,' I shouted across the bar area to where my mum was standing. I ran back and we threw our arms around each other. She held me so tight I could hardly breathe. But I had to go so I picked up my bags and set off again.

She was crying as I looked back and I made up my mind this was not how my visit would end. I would go through the boarding gate with a smile on my face. As I walked on I realized it was the first time I'd been really alone for months. I'd had Mum looking after me all this time but now I had to be a grown-up again and get back into the real world. I felt terrified as I smiled at my mum but I pulled a silly face then turned round and set off for the long journey to my new home.

10. A Mother's Love

Isabell Carstensen was born in Banff, Scotland, in 1948 and moved to Australia 11 years ago after her marriage to Carole's father broke down. She has since married Ivan, who also has two daughters. They live in Canning Vale, Perth. Isabell works part-time as a book-keeper and part-time caring for the elderly. She says: 'When Carole first told me she had MS I felt helpless. My little girl was ill and nothing I could do would make her better.'

It started with a message on my answerphone from a woman with a foreign accent. All I could make out was the name 'Carole'. I couldn't understand anything else she said and put it down to a wrong number. That night, or rather in the early hours of the morning, the phone rang again and it was Carole. She was in hospital in Rio.

We had no idea what was wrong with her, but she said Craig was on his way to her and I knew that was what she really wanted. Once he had arrived she seemed to relax.

She went back to London and had weeks and weeks of tests. When we spoke she always said that she was feeling better. If I asked Craig, he would say the same. With hindsight, I can see that Craig didn't know what was going on in her mind and I realize that she didn't want to worry me, which is why it came as such a shock when she told me early one morning that she had MS.

It was a brief and very matter-of-fact phone call. Neither of us cried, although I wanted to. I felt a horrible mixture of panic and fear, wondering what this would mean for her. I wanted to be with her, to cuddle her. My little girl was ill and nothing I could do would make her better. I felt helpless, but angry too. Why should this happen to *her*? I put the phone down and cried and cried but I had Ivan with me to comfort me.

I didn't really understand what multiple sclerosis was so I looked in the phone book and called the MS Society's branch in Perth. The woman I spoke to said that MS is difficult to explain as no one can predict what pattern it will take, or what time scale it will follow. She said some people were in wheelchairs within weeks or months of diagnosis. On the other hand, one of their members, now in her sixties, had been diagnosed 40 years before and was only just needing to use a walking stick. She also said something which really gave me hope and that was that positive thinking can help. I thought that Carole could do this, I knew she could.

I worried all the time about Carole from then on but my initial anger didn't last very long. It was replaced by fear for her, worrying about her and a feeling of helplessness. How was she coping? What was she thinking? How much wasn't she telling me? Carole has always been protective of me, even when she was a little girl, and I knew she would try not to worry me by saying she was all right. If only I could see her, then I'd be able to tell what was going on in her mind. We have a strong bond; we can tell by a look what the other one is thinking. As every mother will know, that is a very special kind of love. But Ivan and his partner had recently launched their business and I couldn't afford just to hop on a plane so we had to make do with phone calls.

Then my father died and all I could think about was my mum, how she was feeling, and about my dad. I spoke to Carole and she cried and cried but I didn't fly over to Scotland for the funeral. I had loved my dad so much and deep down I couldn't accept that he was dead. Ivan was working offshore at the time. He wanted to come home to me but I said no, so my mother-in-law came to stay. She had a heart attack the day after she arrived. She died five days after my dad: I had lost two people I loved within days. I didn't worry about Carole or how she was coping because I knew she had lots of support from the people around her. I was trying to deal with everything myself at that time.

My mother came to live in Perth a little while later. I couldn't talk to her about Carole because she didn't know Carole was ill. Carole felt that she didn't need to know and I think she was right. But Mum became homesick for Scotland after several months and I took her home. That was a difficult week for me: I was facing my first visit to my dad's grave, I was worrying about leaving Mum and I was trying hard not to show Carole how I was feeling. I cried a lot that week but never to anyone, always on my own. Ivan is my support when I really need it but on the whole I'm someone who requires time to work things out alone.

By then I had really tried to shut the thought of Carole having MS out of my mind. I thought if I didn't talk about it, then it would go away. So neither Carole nor I talked about it and the subject *did* go away. I had been longing to see her, although of course I had so many other things on my mind at that time. But I remember her seeming very tired one evening and watching her try to stay awake to watch TV with Craig. So I said: 'I'm going to bed. I think you look ready for sleep too, Carole.' We looked at each other and I knew that she realized I understood her need to rest.

When I came home to Perth we carried on as usual, phoning every other week. I am the same with both my daughters; I miss them more than anything else and there are times when I need to speak to them. We all need to feel close to one another. I still believe, to be honest, that one day they will come to live in Australia. I imagine them living near me, having a family and visiting all the time. Having a grand-child would be my idea of heaven! But the period after Carole was diagnosed was hard on all of us. What could I do on the other side of the world? I just had to make sure Carole knew I was here for her, and learn as much as I could about MS.

In the end it wasn't her MS which caused a crisis but her boyfriend leaving her. She'd been here with us for Christmas and a couple of weeks later she called me. She was crying so much that I could hardly understand what she was saying. Craig had left her for someone else. My first thought was: 'No, he wouldn't do that to her.' He and I had always got on very well. I thought he was wonderful and had been so happy that he was always there for Carole. I never had any doubts that they loved each other.

But that turned to anger when I realized how much he had hurt my daughter. If he had been anywhere near me at that time I would have hit him. I was concerned about how Carole would cope with the hurt. I knew we needed to be together on this one and I felt she should be here, away from it all. We spoke every day on the phone and I was getting more and more worried about her. Then she rang to say she'd be coming out. It was exactly a month since she'd left us.

When she arrived at Perth airport I remember clearly how she looked when she walked through the arrivals gate. She was smiling that beautiful smile of hers and my heart felt as if it would burst. Then she saw me and just crumbled; she put her hands over her face and sobbed. There was no way I wasn't going to get to her. I pushed my way through all the crowds of people, went under the barrier and held her in my arms. I kept telling her she was all right, she was here now, everything would be all right.

It felt so good having her with me so that I could look after her. She was very tired but I woke her up each morning as usual to get her accustomed to the time difference as quickly as I could. I wanted her to take one day at a time. For the first week she worried a lot about her MS. I think the first turning point came when we had a long talk sitting outside one evening. At last I told her how I felt about the MS and my panic at the thought of her being ill when there was nothing I could do about it. I would imagine every mother wanting to prevent such a thing happening to their child. But MS isn't a grazed knee, and I was utterly helpless. That was a really hard fact to accept.

I knew by then that not talking about MS wouldn't make it go away. I had been wrong to even think like that. But at least I could help her to deal with it, learn to live with it and fight it. She had love and support in abundance as far as I was concerned. But it would be up to her to learn to be happy again.

I think that from then on my daughter began to fight for what she wanted and it was good to see her doing that. I felt really proud of her. She slowly started to look much better and seemed happy again. She made new friends and enjoyed her life here. My cousin, Helen, came to stay with a friend and that meant Carole always had company

– she went shopping, to the beach and generally relaxed and had a good time. Nobody looking at Carole would think there is anything wrong with her and that's true today, too. I could understand when she explained to me how easy it was to lie about her illness. I have learnt to tell now when she is having a bad day. For one thing she doesn't talk so much which, I can assure you, is unusual for Carole!

That visit really gave us the time to talk things through and get back on track. She had new friends, as I said, and my sister got married while Carole was here, but above all she really healed here. She always looks better at the end of a visit than when she arrives. I think by the end of her three months with us she had stopped missing Craig but she wanted someone to take his place in her heart. I did tell her that if ever she decided to go back to him, I would support her decision. By that time I didn't feel it would be a good idea as she would never be able to trust him again. For that reason alone, I felt it wouldn't work.

The day she left to go back to London was the hardest goodbye we've ever had. From the moment I woke up I thought: 'She's leaving today'. At the airport I didn't want to let her go. I'm sure when people talk about their heart breaking that it really does, my heart hurt. For weeks afterwards I kept wishing she'd be there, waiting for me when I came home from work.

I have grown to be very proud of the way Carole copes with her illness. She understands how she feels and knows what to do about it. She has the strength to deal with everything it throws at her. Her attitude does make it easier for me. Had she been the kind of person to give up on it, then I can't imagine how I would feel – particularly with me in Australia and her in London. That really would be a difficult situation to face.

Ivan and I talk about Carole, of course. We agree that MS has changed Carole in that she can't always do as much as she used to, but her personality has stayed the same. She has kept that bubbly, lively attitude which has always made her the centre of attention. Her illness has obviously made her more aware of what can happen in life. I find it important to have time alone with her to discuss everything.

We have to make that time when we see each other, no matter who else is around. My stepdaughters were young when they first found out that Carole was ill, and I still feel they don't really understand the illness, but they've coped very well. They're always interested in what she's doing but they don't dwell on the MS.

At first I didn't tell people – except family and close friends – that my daughter had MS. That was because I wasn't talking about it, anyway. Being able to tell others was a long time coming, partly because I found it hard to accept that Carole was ill. I still do, but at least the two of us talk about it now as we've found that it helps to communicate.

Most people I tell react with shock or surprise. They don't really understand what the illness is. I can understand that because I didn't know at first, either. People are interested to learn about it, and are sympathetic. The first point I make is that she looks well and fit. I think it's because I need to let them know she is doing well. A lot of people feel that I must dread Carole ending up in a wheelchair, but I can't think like that and I know Carole doesn't, either.

We talk regularly on the phone and I always know what is happening with her now. I don't think we'll ever go back to the days when we didn't talk about the MS. I really don't have fears for Carole in the future, I have hopes for her, just as I have hopes for my other daughter, Hazel. I have always been proud of both my daughters. I truly believe that Carole will meet a wonderful man who will love her, look after her and make her very happy.

I think back to how she thought as a teenager; that you meet a tall, dark and handsome millionaire and live happily ever after! Real life isn't quite like that. What she wants and needs now is someone who will be loving, gentle and kind, someone who will communicate with her and who she can depend on, no matter what happens. I want her to have the kind of love and happiness I have found with Ivan, who is the best husband in the world. She still has her hopes and dreams and I believe she will fulfil them. I never gave up on mine and I don't think she will, either.

Of course, there is a lot about her illness that I find disturbing. But if I thought about all the things that could happen then I don't think I'd be a great help to her, and I couldn't cope with that. *What if* she had a relapse and ended up in a wheelchair? *What if* she needed full-time care? *What if* she remained on her own and didn't meet someone to love and care for her? Well, if all the 'what ifs' happen then we will cope with them all.

There have been millions of people in the world who have been thrown into a similar situation, but they don't all give up on life. No matter what happens, I would want my daughter near me. When I asked Ivan what we would do if Carole needed full-time care, he said: 'She would be here with us.' That says it all.

All I would say to any other mum who finds herself in my situation is, don't try and ignore the fact that your child is ill. Talk to them, learn to understand what is happening to them, be there for them when they need you. And, most importantly, don't ever let them give up.

11. A New Beginning

Everything was new when I came home to Britain. It was springtime and that suited my mood. I went from the airport straight to my new home in Wimbledon where my new flatmate, Julie, was waiting for me. I was exhausted and jet-lagged, but determined to see the last three months as a fresh start, a new beginning.

'Carole, you look fantastic!' Julie came running down the path of the Victorian terraced house she had rented for us while I was away.

'Welcome home. Come in, let me help you with those bags.'

I walked in to a pretty living-room with soft cream walls, pale yellow sofas, chintz curtains and a fireplace with a huge mirror hanging above it.

'Julie, it's perfect.'

I looked around, wondering whether I was going to be happy here. I needed to gather my own bits and pieces which I'd given to various friends for safekeeping. My elephant statue, my soapstone ornaments, things I had treated myself to on trips over the past few years. At the moment, it was just somebody else's home, but I had a good feeling about this house.

'Come and see the garden,' Julie said as she led me through the French windows of the dining-room and on the way I glimpsed a tiny kitchen. Hardly room to swing an omelette pan but I was single now. I didn't need to cook every day if I didn't want to. I could do anything I liked.

The tour of the house ended in my bedroom.

'I made up your bed for you,' Julie said as I stared at the sheet and duvet cover she had lent me. I had given my old bedding to a friend. There were to be no reminders of Craig here. I'll buy a new set tomorrow, I thought, in white broderie anglaise. I realized with a start that I wouldn't have to ask anybody else's opinion from now on. I was my own boss and I could have anything I wanted.

'So tell me everything, Carole,' Julie said as we went back downstairs. 'How was Perth? Did you have a good flight? You must be freezing.'

We sat talking for the rest of the afternoon as I willed myself to stay awake past my Perth bedtime to bring my body back to British time. Eventually I gave in and went to bed. I lay with my eyes open in my new room, growing accustomed to the light from the street lamp outside as it threw patterns across the dressing table and in a straight line to the door. My bags were piled in one corner, still with the airline tags on their handles.

How different I felt now than when I'd packed them in January on my way out to Australia. I knew I looked different; tanned, slimmer, fitter. But the biggest difference was inside, the bit nobody could see. From now on I wanted to be upfront about everything and I wanted the same in return. If people asked me about my illness, I'd tell them. I didn't want to become a medical bore but nor would I pretend anymore.

I also had to accept what had happened to me. I had multiple sclerosis and there was no cure. It was my job now to learn to live with it. As I lay there feeling so healthy, it was easy to promise myself that I wouldn't waste a single minute of my life from then on. But I knew the unpredictability was the hardest burden to bear. Would I be all right in the morning? Would I have a relapse during the night? What sort of relapse would my next one be?

If I could learn to live with those fears, to keep them in a compartment at the back of my head so they didn't spoil my day-to-day life, that would be a real achievement.

I went to see my doctor as she and the BA medical staff would need to pass me fit for work.

'Carole, you look absolutely wonderful.'

'A long holiday was the best medicine I could have had.'

'Are you ready to go back to work?'

'I can't wait.'

I had been lucky that people had made the right decision on my behalf when I'd been at my lowest in January. Thank goodness they'd had the wisdom to sign me off work for three months to get the rest I'd needed. Now I had to carry on the good work.

First I would learn to listen to my body. My holiday in Perth had taught me that if I treated my body well, it repaid me by feeling better. From then on a warning symptom would mean that I must rest. No more working like a lunatic to forget. No more ignoring the signs that meant I needed time to myself. And no more anger because I had MS. It was a question of harnessing my energy for the big fight. I'd had my health taken away from me and now it was time to claw back as much of it as I could.

One more thing – I needed BA to give me the all-clear for work.

I was walking down the corridor of Speedbird House at Heathrow airport a few days later when I saw Dr Bagshaw coming towards me. I'd just arrived for my appointment with him and was thinking about his blackboard sketch of a cup spilling over with the stresses of life. That was the last time he had seen me. Would he pass me fit to fly or not? He nodded, said hello to the nursing sister standing next to me and walked on.

'Aren't you speaking to me, Dr Bagshaw?' I shouted after him. He turned and looked at me closely for a few seconds.

'Good grief, it's Carole! You're ... you're *glowing*!'

'It's amazing what a suntan can do.'

'Come with me, Carole, we've got an appointment haven't we?'

I had been an absolute wreck the last time I was in his office. Now I looked like anyone would after three months off work, in the sun, being pampered by their mum. I wasn't with him for long.

'You're ready to go back flying, Carole,' he said with a smile. 'I'm glad it's good news.'

Good news? This was the best, best, best thing. I left his office grinning and practically skipped down the corridor out to my car.

It seemed right somehow that the day I went back to work was the day British Airways launched their Paul Costelloe designer uniform for cabin crew. As we walked through Schipol airport in Amsterdam everyone stopped to stare.

'It's these hats,' I said feeling the top of my unfamiliar red and grey trimmed bowler. I'd been surprised at how nervous I was feeling on my first day back. I could do without people staring and pointing. 'They're all looking at our hats!' I hate my hat to this day, but what can I say? I'm paid to wear it.

It can be frightening to have total freedom but that's what I had. I wanted to learn to be single again. What had I done before I met Craig? For one thing I'd been a party animal, so that summer I fell back into my old habits. But this time round I was a party girl with MS and I'd back out if I had any hint of symptoms. It was no great loss, although I hated the thought of missing a really good one.

'So how was it?' I'd ask friends the next day.

'It was crap, Carole. Honestly, you didn't miss a thing!'

'Yeah, right!'

I thoroughly enjoyed the parties I did go to. I had nobody assuming I would be the driver and nobody dictating when we should go home. Heaven! I was a free spirit again and it felt good. Recovering afterwards took a little longer, but what were a few extra hours in bed if I'd had a good time?

It was very different living with Julie, too. She is more sensible than I am. Her job as a nursery teacher in Knightsbridge and my flying meant we were little more than ships that passed in the night, like most flatmates. But she seemed to know when I was slowing down. I felt comfortable telling her when I was feeling unwell. It was a relief that somebody was listening.

'Shall I run you a bath, Carole? You're looking a bit tired,' she asked one evening as I sat in the living-room, flicking through a magazine but feeling exhausted. I'd had a busy day at work and the old familiar tingling was running up and down my legs.

'Cheers, Jules. That would be great. I think I'll have an early night.' As I went upstairs it struck me that Craig had never once said anything like that. Was he blind? He must have noticed when I was having a bad day. It felt so different to be sharing a house with someone who made the effort to understand.

I made a quick trip down to Somerset to pick up the stuff I'd left at my dad's when I had packed up my flat in such a hurry. Things were very different for him now. He had moved from Devon and remarried. My stepmother, Helena, was only a couple of years older than me. It had taken me a little time to warm to the idea but Helena had won me over. She was such fun, very outgoing. She made Dad happy, so I was happy too. Things had changed a lot in my life recently but that was no reason for everyone else's to stand still.

One thing I never did during that time was go to my doctor. I didn't see the point; they're trained to make people better and no one could do that for me, so why waste their time? I'm not saying that was the right attitude, but it's how I felt. Listening to my body seemed to be working for me.

I started to enjoy my job again, just like the early days when I had first joined British Airways. I was full of energy, too, and that helped. I was ready for the people I worked with to know about my illness; no more putting it off or lying. But I discovered that most people found it impossible to believe that I had MS.

'You're joking, Carole, you look so healthy,' one stewardess said to me when I'd been telling her about MS. We were just coming in to land at Heathrow and I looked down the length of the plane from my seat at the front of the cabin before I answered.

'That's part of the problem,' I said. 'Nobody believes me because that's how MS is a lot of the time. But if I'm not well, then I'm not at work.'

She made me think, though. I felt I was on some sort of private awareness campaign and was finding that most people didn't know what MS was. How could I make the point that you can have MS and look perfectly healthy? I would have to give it some thought.

One thing that was visible was a rash on my chin and top lip which wouldn't go away. Nasty as it was, that rash brought me yet more help in dealing with MS. I was on a trip to Istanbul and was overjoyed to be working with Denise Rothwell again, the girl who'd introduced me to reflexology.

'Carole, you look brilliant!' We'd gone to my room on the twenty-fifth floor of the crew hotel with another stewardess who wanted to try reflexology. We hadn't seen each other for six months and had a lot of catching up to do. Denise had finished with my feet and I felt wonderfully relaxed. She was just starting on the other girl when suddenly everything went black. A power cut! Help! I flicked on my cigarette lighter but could feel the panic rising. We were stuck in pitch darkness, too scared to speak.

Then, just as our eyes were growing used to the blackness, the lights came on again. Denise looked over to the bed and we all laughed. The other stewardess was still lying down, unable to move because her feet were covered in talcum powder ready for a treatment.

'Denise, you're just the person to ask. This rash on my face, is there anything I can do about it?' I sat down next to the bed so we could all chat while Denise worked.

'It hardly shows, Carole, honestly.'

'I think it's the only thing people see when they look at me.'

'Have you tried homeopathy?'

'No. I wonder if it's worth a go. Perhaps it is.'

'Or there's aromatherapy. That can be good if you're stressed.'

I found a homeopathic doctor when I went home and explained my problem to her. She made up a remedy for me to take and banned coffee and anything with mint in it. The medicine made me feel ill and the rash grew worse and worse. Eventually I went back to her.

'Sometimes with homeopathy you have to get worse before you get better,' she explained.

I gave up; I was already on the alert for MS symptoms. I didn't need to inflict anything else on myself. Lots of friends use homeopathy and swear by it, so perhaps it just wasn't for me. At least I'd tried it.

I hit the jackpot when I dropped in to the Beauty Principles salon up the road from my house and met the owners, Sofie and her sister, Sara. They could have sold me anything at the time because by now

I was desperate. Instead Sofie told me exactly what Denise had said.

'Are you under stress?'

'I have been but I'm OK now.'

'Have you tried aromatherapy? It might help.'

Sofie was right; aromatherapy did the trick. The rash disappeared and from then on I've had regular aromatherapy massages – or at least when I can afford them. The problem with alternative medicine is the cost. It's still considered a luxury in this country. I see it as a necessity and wish it could be available on the National Health Service. I know it has helped me and I've learnt to tailor my treatments according to my cash flow. If I'm broke, I'll have a back massage. If I'm in the money, I'll have a full body massage! The next time I bumped in to Denise on a flight I told her I'd been converted. She was delighted.

'Now all you've got to do is stop smoking, Carole.' She laughed and shook her finger at me like a teacher telling off a naughty schoolgirl.

'One thing at a time, Denise. I'll get round to it soon.'

It was a glorious summer so I could keep my Australian tan topped up. I knew I was feeling well because even the heat wasn't affecting me like it had recently. One afternoon Julie and I sat in our back garden, soaking up the sun.

'Isn't it nice having a garden?' Julie said, lying back in the sun lounger as I sprayed myself with the garden hose to cool down.

'It's not like Australia, though,' I said, 'no swimming pool.'

The next evening she came home from work and shouted through the house. 'Carole, where are you? I've bought you a present.'

I walked in from the garden and found her in the kitchen.

'Here you are, Carole, a little bit of Australia for you!'

It was a toddler's paddling pool and I spent hours sitting cross-legged in it, tanning and keeping cool. It was heaven.

One evening I arrived home from work at seven-ish feeling wide awake and full of energy when a friend rang.

'There's a group of us going to a club in Wandsworth, Carole. Do you fancy coming?'

I tore up the stairs flinging bits of my uniform everywhere and was ready in minutes. A few hours' clubbing was just what I needed, then home fairly early for a good night's sleep and a weekend off. When I reached the club I met up with friends and joined a group of students from Zurich who were studying at a college nearby. One of them, Daniella, was really excited. 'There's a male group coming on tonight. I've seen them before. The blond one's really cute.'

'I've never seen male strippers. It's not really my scene.'

But I was bowled over when they came on stage: The Untouchables were five gorgeous guys who also managed to be funny and entertaining. There was nothing tacky about their act. I thought they were fantastic.

'Carole, would you do me a favour?' Daniella looked at me when the group had finished their act. 'I want to meet them, well the blond one, anyway. Will you come with me? Please, please.'

I went hunting for a security guard and asked him whether Daniella could go to the guys' dressing-room to meet them.

'They said they'll see you when they've changed, OK?' I told her and retreated to the bar wondering why I'd become involved in all this. Suddenly a fight broke out at the top of the stairs. A girl went flying down the staircase near the dressing-rooms and lay in a heap.

'Daniella, get out. *Now!*' I screamed across to her as the sound of fighting broke out all around. She made a run for it. I could see that the girl on the staircase hadn't moved and fought my way through the crush to reach her. She was moaning quietly and I leant over her, steadying myself with my outstretched hands against the wall. It was the only way I could protect her. Then I was whacked in the back with a force that took my breath away.

'Oh great, this is all I need. I know one thing, I'm never coming back to this dump again.' I was talking to myself, wondering what to do next. I had to get this girl out of harm's way, although she shouldn't really be moved.

'Call an ambulance, quick!' I shouted at a guy running past. Someone else helped me move the girl into a room. The fight was spreading and a man with his eye cut open came in. He sat on a stool looking pale and shaken. Someone, a bouncer I think, barred me from leaving the room.

'The fighting's bad out there. Stay here, it's safer,' he said.

The ambulance took an hour to arrive. The paramedics said the girl I'd been looking after had injured her vertebrae. I was stuck for that hour, during which I discovered that I was in the male group's dressing-room. My legs had started to tingle and I was getting worried. This wasn't doing me any good at all. I'd been full of energy when I had arrived at the club, but I'd had a full day at work, too. I *needed* my sleep these days. I knew how bad I felt if I didn't get it. When the ambulance had gone and things began to quieten down, Daniella's dream man, the blond one, came over.

'I'm Ricky,' he said, handing me his card. 'Come and see us when we're in London again and bring some friends. On the house. I'm sorry about all this. It's not the best meeting, is it?' He grinned.

It was safe to leave by then so I picked my way up the stairs and went home. I was exhausted and my back ached where I'd been hit. Is that the sort of thing that can trigger a relapse, I thought? I didn't have a clue whether a blow would harm me more now I had MS. There was nothing I could do about it; I certainly wasn't going to wrap myself in cotton wool for the rest of my life. It was the first time in weeks that I'd even thought about relapses.

'Hi, Carole. It's Ricky from The Untouchables here.' It was a few nights after the fight and Julie had passed me the phone as I sat in the living room watching TV.

'Ricky! How are you doing?'

'I'm coming down to London for a photo shoot. Do you fancy meeting for a drink?'

We chatted a bit; he was funny and easy to talk to and I heard myself making my excuses before putting down the phone. I looked up to see Julie staring at me, shaking her head,

'Why won't you meet him for a drink? It sounded like you were hitting it off.'

'I don't know. I'm not sure what men in those sorts of groups are like.'

'For God's sake, Carole, go out and have some fun.'

I rang Ricky back. 'Hi, Ricky. That drink? Is it still on offer?'

A week later, I had a lunchtime flight to Amsterdam. I knew it was going to be fun when I saw that Ray Lewis would be in charge of cabin crew for the flight. A white-haired, tall, smart man, it always cheered me up to hear his Cockney voice. 'You all right, Guv'nor?' he had asked as I entered the briefing room that morning.

I chose to work in club class with Ray and as the passengers started to board I stood behind him while he took their coats and hung them up. I wondered how long I could do nothing before he noticed.

'It's all right, mate, you just stand there while I do all the work,' he said after a few minutes.

'OK, Ray. Anything you say.' We both laughed.

Then the singer Cliff Richard came through the cabin door, or Sir Cliff as he had become. I put my arm out and took his coat and he went to his seat in the front row.

'Do you know, she hasn't taken one coat till you came on,' Ray said to him, smiling.

Cliff Richard laughed and rolled his eyes while I went bright red. Then take-off was delayed. The waiting went on and on and as I sat on a crew seat, Cliff caught my eye.

'I might have to sing a song in a minute,' he said, grinning at me. I pulled the aircraft's internal phone from its stand on the wall.

'Feel free!' I held the microphone out to him and giggled.

I was sitting next to Ray as we were coming in to land at Amsterdam.

'I've never asked anyone for an autograph, Ray, but Mum would love it if I got Cliff Richard's for her.'

'Well, you should ask him.'

'Mum and Dad used to play his music in the car when we were children.'

'Go on. I don't think he'd mind.'

As the plane taxied to its stand at Schipol airport, I plucked up the courage to approach the singer.

'I'm so sorry to disturb you, but could I have your autograph for my mum. She thinks you're wonderful.' I blushed. This was breaking the rules, I knew, but it was too good an opportunity to miss.

'You've left it this long before asking?'

'I was too embarrassed.'

'Get me a piece of paper.'

I fetched a landing card and told him that my Mum's name is Isabell, but people call her Issy. He wrote: 'To Issy, Lots of love, Cliff Richard.'

'There, that wasn't so bad, was it?' he said, handing the card back to me.

'No. This will make her day. Thank you.'

'I can't believe you asked for your *mum*.' We both laughed.

Ray Lewis still tells the story to other crew and always ends with the same line. 'That Carole Mackie, she'll only hang up coats for celebrities.' For me, it was wonderful to be well enough not just to get to work each day, but to have the energy to enjoy my work again. It was almost as though the MS had gone away. I was so healthy that some days I forgot I had it.

Julie first saw Ricky on a baking hot day. He came to the house in ripped jeans, stripped to the waist, and I saw her jaw drop as he walked through the door. He became part of the furniture in our house during that summer, almost like having another girlfriend. If he had a modelling assignment in London he would stay with us, at least once a week. One of the things I loved about Ricky was that he knew about my illness almost from the start and really listened when I was talking about it. That was a new experience for me.

It was nice to have male company without the complications of a relationship and that's how it was with Ricky and me. Everyone assumed we were a couple because we went everywhere together, but we weren't. This was another new experience for me: I'd never truly believed that a girl can have male friends but now I was proving it.

If the guys were doing a show in London, I'd go with them. Sometimes they all slept at our house. One morning I came down to find the five of them making me breakfast, squeezing past each other in our tiny kitchen. Then the phone rang.

'Hello, sweetheart.' It was my dad. No father would understand that his daughter could be perfectly safe with five men in the house at 9.30 in the morning. I put my hand over the receiver.

'Guys, it's Dad. Keep the noise down. I'll never explain you lot to him!'

They all tiptoed around, exaggerating their movements, as I tried to keep a straight face. Later, when they were leaving, I stood at the front door like Snow White as each one gave me a peck on the cheek. The image was shattered as they all climbed into their car, shouting: 'You were great last night, Carole!' A few months before I'd have panicked. What would the neighbours think? These days I didn't care. I was having fun and at last I could be myself. I was still laughing as their car disappeared at the end of the road.

Nobody ever spoke to me about Craig. I kept all the letters I'd written to him in Perth in a fake Louis Vuitton vanity case which I'd bought for next to nothing in Bangkok. It seemed fitting, somehow. On a night stop to Zurich I stayed in a new hotel, out of town and surrounded by mountains. It was peaceful, the only sound the clang of cowbells from a herd of cattle grazing in a field outside my window. I sat down and wrote my final letter to Craig.

'Dear Craig,

Yet another letter you'll never see but this time it's to say goodbye. I've discovered there is life without you, and I'm loving every minute of it.'

I took the letter home and locked it firmly away in the box.

'Carole, do you mind if my agent and his girlfriend come round tonight?' Ricky said one evening when I was feeling shattered.

'I'm knackered, Ricky.'

'Oh go on, they're great.'

I was just finishing the washing up when Paul and Maxine arrived. Paul and Ricky disappeared to discuss work.

'So what do you do, Maxine?' I asked as I was putting away the clean dishes.

'Well, I work as a PA, but I'm studying to be a psychotherapist. I do counselling, too.'

'Really? Now that's something that interests me.' We clicked immediately and before long the subject of MS came up.

'I've done the bit where I didn't talk about it. Now I do talk about it.'

'That's where counselling can be useful,' she replied. 'It can teach people to talk about things.' There was a pause. 'You know, Carole, I was too tired to bother coming out tonight. But I'm glad I did.'

Maxine is now one of my closest friends.

By the autumn I was beginning to calm down. I wasn't scared of being single any longer and I was quite happy with my own company. My need to party endlessly and be busy was wearing off. I was happy being at home. Julie and I might rent a video, or we'd have friends round. Things were becoming normal for me again. I had made some good friends, learnt the value of exploring alternative treatments and thought I'd conquered my fear of telling people that I had MS. Then I met David.

David was a very good-looking New Zealander, easy to talk to, with a good sense of humour, quite wealthy too! But by our third date I still hadn't told him I had MS. When should I tell him? I'd thought about all of this in Australia; it had seemed cut and dried then. In practice it was a lot harder to find the right moment. One evening he took me out for dinner and gave me just the opening I needed.

'A friend of mine's just gone into hospital,' he said.

'Oh no, nothing serious is it?' This was the chance I'd been waiting for. I could easily slip from hospital talk to telling him about my MS.

'No. Well, nothing to worry about. I'll visit him in the next few days. Find out the details.'

Go on, Carole, do it now. I could feel a sense of panic growing and I shifted around in my chair. I felt so uncomfortable. For goodness' sake, do it.

'I'd like a coffee, David. How about you?'

The moment had passed and my fling with David dwindled away.

We stopped seeing each other and he never knew my big secret. I felt relieved. The pressure of not telling him had ruined our time together for me. The best restaurant in London couldn't take my mind off my big secret. I knew I'd never go through that again. After all, what's the worst that can happen? A man could make his excuses not to see me again – and if that was the response, he wasn't a person I'd want in my life anyway. The bottom line was: this is me. If you don't like it then go and I'll carry on with my life.

A few weeks later, just before Christmas, Ricky came over to see Julie and me. He had so much work in London by now that he was living with Maxine and Paul. We were all sharing a huge tub of Cookies and Cream ice cream and watching a video of the Tom Cruise and Jack Nicholson movie, 'A Few Good Men'. One of the characters kept saying: 'You can't handle the truth.' It made me think of David.

'Do you think David would have handled the truth if I'd told him about my MS, Ricky?'

'I didn't know the guy.'

'What would you want a girlfriend to do?'

'Tell it to me straight. Get it right out in the open, Carole. It's the only way. If they can't handle it, that's their problem.'

'It's easier said than done, though.'

'Well it shouldn't be, not if you're with the right person.'

Later in the evening Ricky said: 'I think The Untouchables should do something for charity.'

'Why not do it for multiple sclerosis?'

'Yeah, that's a really good idea.'

'All I need is to find a venue and take it from there.' I could hardly believe what I was saying. Organize a charity event? Where would I begin? 'You could perform with us, just as a one-off. Shock people. Do something they wouldn't expect someone with MS to do.'

'Yeah, right.' We both burst out laughing.

'I'll put it to the guys, Carole. I like the idea.'

The next week, Ricky was back in London.

'You never told the guys, did you Carole?' he said. 'I gave them your idea and they said: 'Great, but why for MS?' I said it's because you've got it. They were stunned. I had no idea they didn't know.'

The job of telling people was obviously more of a problem than I had realized. Then Dad asked my sister and me to spend a weekend with him in Somerset.

We were sitting in the dining-room at breakfast when the phone rang. Dad answered it and passed it to his wife.

'It's for you, Helena.' Dad, Hazel and I were clearing the table and taking the dirty plates into the kitchen when Helena came off the phone.

'Are you two talking baby talk again?' Dad shouted through to Helena, who was standing at the foot of the stairs.

'Oh, is her friend expecting a baby?' I asked him.

'Yes, she is. And so is Helena.'

Hazel and I leapt at Dad and threw our arms around him. By the time Helena came into the kitchen we were all crying. This was such good news. I had never dreamt I would have another baby brother or sister at this time in my life.

'We arrived last night, Dad. Why did you wait until now to tell us?' I asked him when we were chatting later.

'I was waiting for the right moment, sweetheart.'

I knew exactly what he meant.

After months of giving off bad signals – Go away, I'm miserable, I hate men – I now felt so happy that it was as though everyone wanted to be with me. If only I could have three months off every year. That long rest had given me back my normal lifestyle. In fact, I could forget some days that I had MS. I was free to do what I liked and was open to having fun again. I was treating my body well and it was repaying me by staying well. It's amazing what a difference your attitude really does make.

Now I had another challenge on my hands. How would I organize a charity event? I'd never done anything like that in my life and I was scared. Not only about putting an event together. If I went ahead, my illness would become public property and I wasn't sure how I would react to that. Total strangers would be able to say: 'There she is, that's the girl with MS.' I had two choices: I could back out or brave it out.

12. Going Public

'Carole, it's great to hear from you. What are you up to?' I had spent Christmas thinking over the charity event and had decided to take the plunge. Phoning Neil Fox seemed a good place to start.

'I want to pick your brains. I'm thinking of organizing a fundraising event for multiple sclerosis. What do you think?'

I had known Neil for years and now he was Capital Radio's star DJ, Dr Fox, making lots of public appearances all over London. Surely he'd know about these things?

'It's a good idea. Have you found a venue?'

'No, but I was thinking of somewhere big, like the Hammersmith Palais.'

'No, that's too big. You need somewhere smaller so you can pack it out. It creates a better atmosphere. People will want you to do another one!'

'Mmm. I'm not sure. I find it scary, to be honest.'

'You're perfect for this, Carole. You'll be great. How about somewhere like Stringfellows? It holds about 600 to 700 people, I think. Why not give them a ring?'

'One last thing, Neil. Would you come along to it?'

'OK, I'll be your DJ. I can advertise it on my radio show, too.'

'The only problem is, you won't get any money.'

'Carole, what are friends for?'

I put down the phone with a lump in my throat. His support meant a lot to me.

The next morning I plucked up the courage to phone the club. I was put through to the manager, Mary Daws.

'That all sounds fine, Carole. Can you make it on one of our less busy nights, say a Tuesday or Wednesday? Now what dates do you have in mind?'

Slow down, I thought. It's only January. Can't I put off naming a date for a while?

'I haven't set a date yet, Mary. Can I come back to you?'

'What are you waiting for? You've got an event. All you need now is a sponsor for tickets and posters. Give me a call when you're ready.'

The next few weeks passed in a frenzy. I phoned the MS Society for the first time and they put me in touch with my local branch at Merton – I didn't even know the Society had local branches. Their welfare officer, Claire Taylor, became my right-hand woman. It was going to be all right: I could see the point of doing all this once I had decided that the money we raised would help projects that the Merton branch supported.

I went to my father's for a weekend and told him about the event. 'So all I need now is a sponsor.'

'You'd better start writing to companies, Carole. You don't have much time. We get lots of letters but we need notice to organize everything.'

'How do you know all about it?'

'I'm on the sponsorship committee at work.'

Dad worked for Taunton's Cider and they agreed to be my sponsors. Within a couple of weeks I was sitting with him, his sales team and Mary Daws at Stringfellows. It was a baptism of fire.

'So, Carole, how many tickets do you plan to print?'

'Seven hundred.'

'Yes, but how many people do you think will actually bother to come?'

'At least six hundred.'

'I'm just concerned about how many we need to cater for, realistically. Some people will buy tickets then not go along on the night.'

I tried to see myself through their eyes. I had no track record. I was a stewardess, what did I know about this sort of thing? But I was convinced, somehow, that it would be a success. I was relieved when the meeting ended.

'Well, sweetheart, it was nice doing business with you.' Dad shook my hand as we left the room. This event was already forcing some changes within me. A few weeks before, I would have said he and I were both too headstrong to sit round a table at a business meeting and reach an agreement!

The pieces of the jigsaw were beginning to fit. British Airways donated two tickets to anywhere in the world for the raffle, the MS Society's press officers drummed up a few celebrities – Nicholas Parsons and *Coronation Street's* Chris Quentin, among others – and all that was left for me to do was the publicity.

Then I fell sick. Good old MS. Just when I was putting my heart and soul into something, it slapped me down. I felt exhausted. It was such a shock after months and months of being healthy but all I could do was stay at home and rest. At least I could use the phone. I rang BA's staff magazine, *Contact*.

'Of course we'll give you some publicity, Carole. What date is your event?'

Then my father rang.

'We need to print the posters, sweetheart. Have you set a date yet?'

I plucked 23 May, 1995 out of the air.

'By the way, Carole, can you send us a photograph of yourself for our article about your charity event?' The woman at the BA magazine made it sound like the most natural request in the world.

I thought long and hard that day. By the evening I had written a long piece for the magazine with all the details they needed. I made it personal, told some of my own story, and gave it to my flatmate Julie to read. Ricky had come to see us and he looked it over, too. I was unsure about taking this step, but they loved it and I posted it off – without a photograph. A lot of people at BA already knew that I had MS but I was terrified of going public at work. I wasn't ready to be singled out as different. So when Ricky mentioned his idea again my decision didn't make much sense.

'Carole, it would be brilliant if you came out and danced the first bit of our act with us. Have you given it any thought since we talked about it before Christmas?'

Ricky still wanted me to perform with The Untouchables on the night of the event. I was half hoping he'd forgotten the idea!

'We'll keep it secret. You could tuck your hair up into a baseball cap or something. One of us will drop out and you'll take their place. You can wear our gear. No one will know until you take your hat off!'

'No way, Ricky. I've seen the dance routine. I can't do that.'

'Look, Carole. You'd be making an important statement: That someone with MS can do it. People won't expect it. While you're resting, sit and watch our routine on video. Then I'll teach you what to do.'

Which is how, a few weeks later, Ricky and I were in the dance studio of my local health club with 'Bad To The Bone' blaring out as he took me slowly through the steps of The Untouchables' opening routine. Some bits were too raunchy for me. I had to put my foot down.

'I am not thrusting my pelvis for anyone, Ricky!' I was laughing over the music.

My legs were in agony after the rehearsal but they were the least of my worries. There would be 600 people watching – and my dad would be among them. He'd die from shock when he realized what his daughter was doing. But he would know it was for a good cause.

The staff magazine article was published in March and I was nervous about going in to work. I wondered whether cabin crew would be thinking: 'I don't want to fly with Carole Mackie now that I know she's got MS. What if she can't cope in an emergency?' The only comparison I could think of was coming out of the closet. It's well known that a lot of air stewards are gay and some had described to me the unexpected reactions they had faced when they broke their news to colleagues. Now it was my turn.

I'm not sure how I survived that day at work. Our mail is collected for us in drop files and I couldn't get to mine until the afternoon. I walked over to it trembling and before I reached the file I could see it was bulging with letters, notes, pages torn out of notebooks. I glanced at several.

'Dear Carole, I just wanted to say how brave I think you are ...'

'Dear Carole, I've worked with you all the years since you were diagnosed and I never once knew that you had MS. Please let me know if there's anything I can do to help. I'll see you at the event ...'

I scooped up the file and drove home. I sat at the dining table and spread the letters out in front of me. I had read only a few before the tears started. Every single letter was supportive, whether from people I knew or strangers I had never worked with. They all wanted tickets for the event and I no longer had any fears about organizing it. I knew that with their strength behind me, I couldn't fail. It was also another weight off my shoulders. The fear of people finding out accidentally that I had multiple sclerosis had been awful. Now all of my colleagues knew, not just the few I had spoken to over the past few months since I had started to be more open. Their letters showed that all they wanted to give me was support and understanding.

I realized that my decision to begin fund-raising was going to teach me things about my illness I had never confronted before. For the next month I did interviews with local newspapers and even the paper in Banff, Scotland, where I'm from. Then I opened a copy of *Skyport*, Heathrow airport's own newspaper. The headline used the phrase 'MS victim' and I was described as a 'sufferer'. I was furious. It all sounded so negative, not how I felt at all. So I rang the reporter to tell her so. But as I was talking to her I realized that it was part of my job to educate people not to use these labels. I don't want anyone thinking of me as a victim, but unless I tell them that's how I feel they won't know. Another lesson had been learned the hard way.

I was chatting to Maggie Sheppard, my performance manager, one day. 'How are you feeling, Carole?' she asked.

'I'm fine, just a bit tired.'

'I'm proud of what you're doing, Carole, but do look after yourself, won't you? Perhaps you're attempting too much.'

She was right. I was working full-time and organizing the event, but I'd never felt so determined in my life. This was going to be a success.

A week before the event Kingston FM, my local radio station, wanted to interview me. Their breakfast show presenter, David Mason, rang me and was very reassuring.

'You'll be fine, Carole. Just behave naturally and you'll forget we are on air.'

'How many people listen?'

'About 50,000. I'll see you in the morning.'

I arrived at the Teddington Studios at 8.30 a.m. and David's reassurances of the night before evaporated.

'You'll be on air for 40 minutes, just join in the conversation and don't worry about a thing,' David said, no doubt thinking that was a comfort.

When the red GOING LIVE sign began to flash above my head I thought I was going to be sick. But I wasn't and it was fine and I learnt two more things. Firstly, on radio if you don't like a question you have been asked you can give the presenter a look and the listener is none the wiser. Secondly, I didn't know as much about this illness of mine as I'd thought.

'So, Carole, how many people in the UK have multiple sclerosis?'

I had to wave my hands and shake my head. I had no idea what the answer was and I needed him to move on to safer ground. It was time I started to educate myself properly about this thing that was changing my life so dramatically.

I had never learnt to delegate jobs. Well, I'd never really needed to and I'm the type of person who wants to do everything myself, to be certain it is all right. Friends were selling tickets for me but I was running around like an idiot and as the date drew nearer there seemed to be more and more to do.

The night before the event I arrived home from work to find my answer phone flashing with messages. I checked my mobile phone and that had a string of calls to answer, too. They were all last-minute hiccups. I had to escape, to clear my head, so I went for a walk on Wimbledon Common. I sat on a bench, staring at the grass, soaking up this chance to be alone. Then I made my way home.

'Carole, you look really tired,' Julie said kindly. I burst into tears.

'I am. I can't believe how much there is to do.'

'You need a good rest tonight.'

'I feel so nervous. What if it's a flop? What if something goes wrong?'

'Everything will be fine. Why don't you have a bath while I cook dinner?'

'And while you're in the bath I'll deal with all these telephone calls. OK?' Ricky smiled at me from the sofa and I went upstairs.

The three of us had just finished eating when Neil Fox rang.

'Carole, get your tape recorder running, I'll be talking about your event in 10 minutes' time. Can't stay. Bye.'

I switched on the radio and put a blank tape in the recorder, turning up the volume as Neil's programme began. A few minutes into his show, the music stopped and Neil's voice came on.

'Tonight I would like to tell you about a friend of mine and how she is dealing with something that has changed her life ...'

By the end I was speechless. I hadn't realized he would make his appeal so personal. I looked at Julie and Ricky. None of us spoke. I walked over to stop the tape recorder and as it clicked off, the atmosphere broke.

'Carole, it's time to brush up on our dance routine,' Ricky said. 'Here you are.'

He handed me the video remote controller and put the TV on.

'Just keep watching. It's the best way to remember it.'

Play, rewind; play, rewind. After about 20 times, I was too tired to think. I went to bed and fell into a deep sleep.

I woke feeling completely relaxed and clear-headed. The phone was still ringing but I didn't mind. I wasn't even nervous when Ricky took me through the dance routine. We were doing it yet again when the BBC car arrived. They had asked me to be on Radio 5 Live's Drivetime programme and the opportunity was too good to miss. As I arrived at BBC Broadcasting House my mobile phone rang.

'Carole, it's the press office at BA. There's been an incident on one of our planes, an emergency operation on a passenger with a coat hanger.'

'You're kidding!'

'They may ask you questions about it on the radio.'

'Well I can't answer them, I didn't even know it had happened till you rang.' I'd been given a dressing-room after I had explained I would need to dash from the studio straight to Stringfellows. I hung my black evening dress on the back of the door, sat down in front of the mirror and began applying my make-up. I wasn't happy with the dress. It wasn't me; it was too revealing. It was a warm evening, but I put a black jacket on over the dress. I didn't have the confidence not to worry about my cleavage all evening! Then I had the call to go to the studio.

I walked along the corridor and caught a sideways glimpse of myself in a mirror. I noticed I hadn't finished putting in my heated rollers. I looked a complete mess. It's radio, Carole, it doesn't matter what you look like, I kept telling myself.

But when I reached the studio I felt calm. I knew why I was there and would do my best. When the words came out of my mouth I barely recognized that it was me speaking.

'I was diagnosed four years ago and I wouldn't be doing what I'm doing now if I didn't have MS,' I said as the presenter John Inverdale introduced me just before the seven o'clock news.

'How did you feel when you first discovered that you had the condition?'

'I was really angry. I thought I would lose my job, that I'd be in a wheelchair and become a cripple.'

'How do your colleagues react at work?'

'They don't feel sorry for me. They are learning from me.'

'Tell us about the party you've organized for tonight, Carole.'

'When I started out, my aim was to raise money for research. Now it has taken a new turn. I want to make people aware of what MS is. I want people to learn from me.'

'Do you see a new challenge ahead after tonight's event is over, Carole?'

'I have lots of things in my head for the coming year. I want people to realize when they are diagnosed that it's not the end, because it isn't. This really is only the beginning for me.'

I walked out of the studio in a daze. Something important had happened to me in the past few minutes. I hadn't planned what I would say in the interview and yet each answer had been exactly how I felt. It was as though a fog had lifted inside my head and I could see everything clearly for the first time since I was diagnosed with MS.

I arrived at Stringfellows ten minutes late and it was already filling up. There were so many people that I recognized – friends, cabin crew whom I hadn't seen for ages. But I couldn't stop to talk with any of them – there was too much to do.

'Carole, you must meet Adam.' I looked up to see Christine, my hairdresser and a friend going back years, in front of me. Adam was her new boyfriend and I'd heard lots about him but hadn't yet met him. Just then Nicholas Parsons came over to introduce himself.

'I'll be with you in a few minutes, Christine,' I shouted over to her. I never did get to meet Adam that night. I was on duty and had lots to do all evening. I couldn't make the time to talk to friends. I found that really hard; it was the first time I'd ever been in that position.

'Carole Mackie, please would you go upstairs.' Neil Fox's voice came over the microphone. I fought my way through the crowd and just as I was dealing with a query at the bar, another message came through. 'Carole Mackie, please would you go to the main reception area.' It seemed that wherever I was, I needed to be somewhere else. Eventually I made my way onto the stage for a word with Neil, who had everyone dancing.

'Neil, if you give out one more announcement for me to go upstairs, downstairs, or anywhere else, I'll hit you!' We both laughed.

'It's going well, Carole.'

Then I heard a girl's voice behind me.

'Are you Carole Mackie, the organizer?'

'Yes, that's right. Hello.'

'It said on the tickets that The Untouchables would appear at 10 p.m. So where are they?'

'I'm sorry, some of them had to drive down from Manchester and they're a bit late. They've arrived now, though, so it won't be long.'

'Well, we've got a bus to catch. We're going to miss them and they're what we came for.'

'I'm really sorry. Look, if you want to see them that badly, why don't you all club together for a taxi?'

'That's not good enough. This is very badly organized.'

She walked off and I felt really hurt. I turned round and Neil was standing there.

'Carole, there are some sad people in the world and you've just dealt with one of them.' He gave me a hug but she had upset me. I wanted everyone to have a really good time. Just then Ricky came up the steps at the side of the stage. I told him what had happened. He put his arm round my shoulder.

'Carole, look around this room. You did this and you should be really proud of yourself. Now let's get changed. It's time for our act.'

'I'll be right behind you.' I gave myself a quiet minute to soak up the atmosphere of the packed club, with hundreds of people having a good time. He was right and I'm glad I have that moment to remember.

'Neil, you'll cover for me won't you?' My act was a secret. Only Neil, Julie and my sister Hazel knew, so if anyone asked where I was while I was getting changed, they'd lie for me. It was Hazel's job to keep my dad – who had come alone as Helena was now too heavily pregnant for the trip up from Somerset – downstairs near the stage so he wouldn't miss the act.

I squeezed into the tiny changing-room with Julie and four of The Untouchables and let them dress me. I didn't know what to do with most of the gear. It was hardly what I was used to; riding boots, black jodhpurs, a military jacket. What had I let myself in for? It was all so hot, too. Sweat was beginning to trickle down the sides of my face. I felt dreadful.

'Look, I'm getting really nervous. Maybe this was a bad idea. I'm sorry,' I announced. I glanced out of the dressing-room door and could see some staff clearing the stage. 'There are too many people out there. I can't do it. What if I make a mistake?' Julie put her arm round my shoulder.

'Carole, if you forget any of the steps, just look to your right, left or straight in front,' Ricky said patiently. 'We'll put you in the middle and you can take your lead from us. You'll be great.'

'I'm wearing *sunglasses* in a nightclub. How can I see what anyone is doing?' Just then Neil Fox's voice came through the crowd.

'Ladies and gentlemen. The Untouchables.'

'Good luck, Carole,' Julie kissed me on the cheek.

The four boys and I walked onto the stage, knelt on one knee like runners starting a race and waited for the music. My heart was beating so hard I could hear it. Then the music exploded and it was amazing. I went straight into the routine, each arm and leg movement coming naturally. The rehearsals had paid off. I didn't make one wrong move and I loved every minute of it. I could hear that the audience was shouting and clapping, but I couldn't see them. I could feel that it was all going well. Then it was over.

As arranged, I walked over to Neil, taking off my sunglasses as I went. I grabbed the microphone from his hand and threw off my baseball cap. As my hair fell loose and people started applauding I shouted out: 'Ladies, these are my boys. Do you want to see more?'

The girls in the audience were screaming by now and began to surge towards the dance floor. As the men disappeared to the bar for a drink The Untouchables carried on with the rest of their act.

All I wanted was to change my clothes and sit down, but instead I had to run upstairs to have my photograph taken with Neil, Dad and his sales team. Then someone else dragged us back downstairs to the stage. Nicholas Parsons made a speech and had everyone roaring with laughter, then my dad gave his thanks. But I couldn't say everything I wanted to, it was too emotional.

I dashed from the stage to the dressing-room and sank onto a hard wooden chair as I pulled off the boots and jodhpurs. I felt so hot and excited as I put on my evening dress again. I looked in the mirror. You're doing OK, I told myself, savouring this time alone with the noise of voices and laughing coming through the walls. I scraped my hair, which looked a mess after being scrunched into a baseball cap, into a pony tail, put on some lipstick, took a deep breath and went back into the crowd.

I walked upstairs to find Peter Stringfellow, and thanked him for the use of his club. Then I told him about the girl who had complained. Despite everything else, that was still playing on my mind. I hated the thought that someone felt let down.

'One complaint out of 600, Carole? Now that's what I call a successful evening!'

He was right, of course. You can't make everyone happy. If I was going to do more fund-raising, I'd have to learn to take complaints as well as compliments.

I walked over to the bar. 'I think you deserve a glass of champagne,' one of the staff said.

'A cup of hot chocolate would be even better.' I eased myself onto a bar stool. My feet were stinging, my legs hurt, I was very tired – and I hadn't been so happy for ages.

'Cheers!' I said as he handed me the hot chocolate.

Soon after, people began to leave. The evening had flown by. Friends have told me that a wedding takes months to arrange then flashes past, and that's how I felt. All that hard work, you click your fingers and it's gone. I hadn't even had time to talk to any of my friends.

But there was one big bonus: we had raised £6,500 just from having a party. With funds the Merton branch had already raised, we would buy a £10,000 piece of equipment which the Institute of Neurology in London needed. What a great feeling that was. I went home almost too tired to walk, but more pleased than I could ever remember.

The next morning I woke up and grinned to myself. Friends kept ringing to congratulate me. It was a good feeling; it had been one of the most worthwhile things I had ever done. I lay on the sofa and realized that now I had nothing to do. I had spent months with a list of phone calls to make or people to see and now it was all over. I put the tape of my BBC radio interview on. It was only the previous night but it seemed ages ago.

'Do you see a new challenge ahead after tonight's event is over, Carole?' The presenter's question boomed through the living-room and I was struck by my voice in reply. It was so quiet, but had a new determination in it that I didn't recognize.

'This is only the beginning.' Where did I get that from? I drifted off to sleep on the sofa.

I was sitting in the staff restaurant at Heathrow about two weeks later, reading a newspaper. I had three hours to kill before my next flight, to Zurich. Then my mobile phone rang.

'You've got a little baby sister!' It was my dad, sounding exhausted but so happy.

'Is Helena OK?'

'She's tired, but she's fine. Everything went well. Nothing to worry about.'

'What have you called her?'

'Abigayle Rebecca Mackie.'

'Abi? Oh, I like that. I can't wait to see her. Give my love to Helena and I'll speak to you when I get back from Zurich.'

The baby was a week old when Hazel, her boyfriend Paul and I made it down to Devon. Abi was perfect. As I looked at her it struck me as strange that Dad had managed to marry and have a baby before me. It wasn't something I'd ever expected. But 1995 was proving to be a good year for me.

Everything changed for me after my charity event. I had been scared every step of the way. Each new experience leading up to it had taught me new things about me and my illness. Now everyone I worked with knew that I had multiple sclerosis. Because I had made contact with the MS Society I began to keep up-to-date with developments in research. I read and read and realized that I was becoming more aware, too. It was my job to educate people about this illness and that was what I would do. I had found my purpose. I didn't know where it would take me, but at long last I had stopped asking: *Why me? I knew, for the first time, why I had MS.*

13. The Father's Story

Ron Mackie was born in Banff, Scotland, in 1947. Since his divorce from Carole's mum he has married Helena and they have one daughter, Abi. Ron now works as a sales director with Matthew Clark plc and lives in Puriton, Somerset. 'You have to consider the burden of looking after someone full-time, but we'll treat that problem when we come to it,' he says.

When Carole was first taken ill I wondered what could be wrong with her. Was it something she ate, or some sort of nervous disorder? While she was in Rio I felt her mother should be the one to go out to her. I was really disturbed and disappointed that she chose to fly Craig out. She is very close to her mother. If anything had happened to her, if she had died, I think I would have felt very bitter knowing that neither of us had been with her.

When she came home to England she described to me some of the exercises she was asked to do before she was finally diagnosed. I remember she had to distinguish between a 10p piece and a 50p piece in her purse, just using her fingers. But she couldn't feel any difference because her fingers were numb.

Multiple sclerosis was the last thing I was thinking of at that stage. I suspected there had to be something fairly seriously wrong otherwise why would she have been in hospital? When she was flying long-haul Carole used to go all over the world. I thought perhaps the continuous time changes and disruption to her system had taken its toll. I remember she simply said: 'I have a form of MS.' I didn't know how many types of the illness there were. We have never really got down to the nitty-gritty details of the illness.

I didn't look up anything about the illness, not because I was afraid of what I'd find out. Neither have I given any thought to finding out about it. I haven't gone into the gory details about what happens, what makes it advance. I don't worry about that.

I have met people with MS and even now, to me, Carole doesn't have it. I have met someone who was in a wheelchair with it, and known of someone else who died. After Carole's first charity event one colleague came up and told me that his wife has MS. Since Carole's diagnosis I have become more aware of other people and their friends and family who have multiple sclerosis. Carole doesn't strike me as having MS because she appears perfectly normal. There is no wheelchair involved, no home help is needed, there are no outwardly visible signs. You have to be around when something does go wrong to be convinced that she really is suffering from the illness.

This happened to me when she was visiting us in Somerset. I was watching a late programme on TV when Carole, very distraught, crying and literally shaking like a leaf came into the living-room. I held her and comforted her till she calmed down. It had started while she was asleep and the shudders through her body had woken her up. I slept in the room next to hers that night. I guess I was concerned there was something seriously wrong with my daughter.

Abi was ill with a severe tummy bug at the time. After a visit to her doctor when she went home, it appeared that Carole had picked up the bug. Because of her MS, the effects of it on her had been different and quite extreme.

Carole gets tired very quickly and sometimes looks absolutely washed out. She talks about her legs tingling and things like that. But I think she pushes herself too hard. She did a tremendous job with her charity events. I don't know or understand where she gets her energy from.

I was a fairly distant father when Carole and Hazel were kids. I married young and would do things differently if I had my life over again. I was a wild character and family life was a very low priority. I was one of the lads and went out and did laddish things.

With my first marriage over and Carole and Hazel grown up, Helena and I were free to do everything and anything before Abi was born. But I knew Helena wanted a baby. Abi is three years old now and picks things up very quickly. If I tried to explain to her that Carole is ill she'd just keep saying to Carole: 'Why are you sick?' I will leave telling her about Carole until she can understand what I am talking about. I told Helena about Carole in the very early days of our relationship. There was no lengthy discussion nor any major issues arising from the subject.

When Isabell (Carole's mum) moved to Australia I assumed Carole and Hazel would move there too. I am delighted but surprised they are here. Carole's job, with its subsidized flights, has been a real bonus for us as a family as it means Carole and Hazel have been able to see their mother regularly.

It bugged me a bit when she was given a car on disability allowance. She has a good job and I didn't understand why she got it. There are people worse off than her. It was like someone with a job claiming unemployment benefit. Again, I felt like this because I thought of Carole as though there was nothing wrong with her.

I knew Carole would cope with MS. Everything is front-on with her. What would really hit her would be a relapse that takes her into the next stage of MS. I don't think she fully understands what it could be like. She doesn't come across as worried about it. She wants to be mobile, the centre of attention. She has great charisma. She could do a number of jobs through the force of her personality alone. I think in recent years she has become more analytical and maybe this illness has made her like that.

Carole and I have always argued; she gets on her high horse and I fly off the handle and we don't see each other for weeks, sometimes months. Up to a certain age we all show bravado about life. I was like that and Carole was, too. Now, though, she plans ahead and thinks around things. Both my daughters are good girls, they are both hard-headed, like their parents. They are like I was at their age; they stand up and fight. I have never allotted more time to Carole because she is ill, although perhaps I do phone her more often, just to check that she is all right.

My side of the family aren't particularly protective towards her because she is ill. They always ask how she is getting on but Carole's

MS hasn't changed how we are as a family. It's not a topic of conversation all the time.

I think Carole has far too high expectations of the man she wants to meet. She wants to marry a millionaire, but then, who doesn't? She can't hide her MS away from men. Most guys would have second thoughts about taking on someone with MS. Maybe not in the early stages, but later they will. She will know when the right man comes along. I liked Craig. He was quiet, a sound guy, but Carole ruled the roost with him too much. It wouldn't surprise me if she met someone who has MS or some other form of illness.

He will have to have the personality and outgoing nature that Carole has, they will have to match. They need parity, otherwise it won't work. Maybe someone will take her on board. But I don't think she will find an Adonis; whoever he is will have to understand and accept all that she is. I wouldn't take on someone with MS, not even if she was Miss World. I know myself too well now, and somewhere down the road things would go wrong. I no longer think there's any sense in trying to make something work if it's basically wrong. She has to find someone soon; underneath, I think she wants a baby.

I think about Carole's MS more now than I used to, perhaps because I'm getting older. Also, because her illness has caused her to do so many different things. Nothing surprises me with Carole. When she gets an idea and immerses herself in it, it's all systems go. She doesn't like things to go wrong. As far as I can see, MS plays no part in her day-to-day life. Neither is it used to influence, negotiate or demand favours.

I do talk about Carole's illness to my friends. I don't bring it up out of the blue, but if someone's seen something on TV or in the papers, then I'll talk. I don't get into deep discussions because I'm not qualified.

I don't think Carole tells me everything. Perhaps she doesn't want to worry me or perhaps she prefers to handle things herself. She'll phone me to say she has to get away. But I don't know whether she is feeling ill or just needs a break from time to time.

Looking into the future, I do worry in case the MS advances. Who will look after her? What can I do? What must I do? I would take one step at a time. I don't know if there would be problems for her getting into Australia if she was ill. I think she would bounce towards her mum rather than me.

I don't discuss all of this with Carole; we have touched the boundaries of it, though. But I have never asked her what she is going to do. I would never say that she must stay in this country. I wouldn't worry too much if she decided to go to her mother. I am 51 per cent in favour of Australia, 49 per cent in favour of her staying in England. She has her friends, contacts and lifestyle here so I'm not sure Australia would be right for her. You have to consider the burden of looking after someone full-time, but we'll just treat that problem when it comes.

What would I say to other fathers in our situation? Firstly, everyone's make-up is different. Each has their own mentality, circumstances, lifestyle, family, financial situation, work – no two people are the same. We would have to ask Carole what she wants. There would be no sense in her mum screaming from one end of the world and me at the other, both wanting her to be with us. I just hope she realizes I will always be here for her and I know I have Helena's full support if Carole wanted to come here.

My advice to others would be to analyze your own situation carefully. Think about the individual and what they want, what you *want* to do and what you can do for them. Enlist all the help you can get from doctors, counsellors, friends and relatives, too. Talking with my sales hat on, it's about preparation and planning, to determine the best outcome for both parties. Like any father I have always wanted the best for my girls. If a cure was found I would do all that I could to get it for her. Beyond that I hope and pray that her condition remains in remission and doesn't deteriorate.

I don't want to see Carole stop flying. I think it's very important that she should stay with British Airways. I hope somewhere in their offices there is a written plan for her. Financial security is the key for her. She needs things in writing, not just promises. I have never flown with Carole but I think her job is perfect for her gregarious and outgoing personality.

I can't see her sitting behind a desk. She is a people person. She'd make a good fund-raising organizer. She needs freedom; she's like a butterfly, a free spirit. Or make that a bee, always buzzing around.

I think Carole copes very well with her illness. I wonder what she thinks when she's alone and locks her door at night. I know I worry about her if I think about her at that time. I am damn sure she is concerned about what the future holds for her. I don't think I see her as anything but a normal person. I wonder sometimes what her colleagues think about flying with her; about whether she'll have a relapse in the air and will they know what to do about it. But to be honest, I bet it never even crosses their minds.

14. My Worst Nightmare

'Are you all right, Carole?' My manager, Maggie Sheppard, spotted me as I made my way to the crew briefing room before a flight to Bilbao, Spain, early one morning.

'I think so, but I've got a really bad stomach ache.' Maggie looked at me, concerned.

'Are you sure you're OK to fly today?'

'Yes, I'll be fine. Don't worry.'

'Well, you know how you feel.'

I felt terrible, truth be known. I'd had a sore stomach for several days and that morning it felt bloated. But it was only a 90-minute flight. Not much could go wrong in that time, surely?

I was on one side of the drinks trolley, serving passengers in club class, and the purser was on the other when a pain shot through my stomach. It was so sharp and so sudden it made me bend over, by instinct, wrapping my arms around my body.

'I need to go to the toilet,' I said quietly to the purser, and she pushed the trolley over to one side of the aisle so I could squeeze past.

I dashed into the toilet, fumbling to lock the door so the light would come on. But I didn't make it on to the loo in time. I couldn't move. I stood frozen, in shock.

Oh my God, what do I do now? I began shaking from head to foot and leant on the sink with both hands, looking down at the mess. I glanced up at the mirror and even in the ghostly light of an aircraft toilet I could see that I was completely drained of colour. Oh no, what is happening to me?

I opened the door very slightly to find the purser standing outside.

'I've had the most terrible accident. I'm so sorry.'

She handed me through some hot towels while I fumbled with my skirt, managing to get it off in the cramped cubicle. I washed it out in the sink, still shaking. The purser passed me a passenger blanket to wrap around myself. It was then that I remembered the toilet was at the front of the plane. I had to walk out, ashen-faced, wearing the blanket as a skirt, *in front of all the passengers.*

'Carole, drink this. It might help.' The purser, a nurse before joining the airline, handed me a piping hot cup of tea. I had made it to the privacy of the galley but I was burning with embarrassment. I could feel tears welling up in my eyes.

'Don't worry, you'll be all right.' She laid her hand on my arm.

Then I started to cry. I felt so ashamed – and frightened. Was this my worst nightmare coming true? I had to put my fear into words.

'What if it's the MS? What if I'm incontinent?' I said, trying to keep my voice as low as possible.

'It might not be. Why don't you sit down? Try not to worry.'

Luckily the flight wasn't full. I shrank into a window seat, trying to make myself invisible. I watched as the purser blocked off the toilet. I wanted to be hundreds of miles away, at home, lying in a hot, sweet-smelling bath. A few passengers stopped in the aisle to ask if I was feeling all right. I stared ahead at the closed toilet and sank and sank further into my seat, humiliated.

We landed at Bilbao and I persuaded the pilots that I didn't want medical attention, I just needed to get home. I stayed on the plane, willing the minutes to pass before we could be on our way. My skirt dried and I put it back on while the poor cleaners tackled the disgusting job of cleaning out the loo. I settled into my window seat feeling weak and shaky. Every now and then a sob would escape. For most of the journey I stared out at the clouds in utter despair.

I was sitting in the nursing sister's office at Heathrow when my manager walked in.

'I'm so sorry, Maggie, I'm so sorry.' I burst into tears again. She had trusted me to tell her how I felt and I'd been wrong. I had broken my side of our bargain – that I would never fly if I was ill.

'My stomach has hurt for ages, but my doctor wasn't on duty when I went to see her. Her locum said I've got irritable bowel syndrome. He gave me some tablets to take if the pain was bad. I should have told you.'

'Don't worry, don't worry. Let me get you a car to take you home.' She put her arm round me.

'I don't want any fuss. I'll drive myself. I just want to have a bath.'

'Are you sure? Let me phone your doctor and get an appointment for this evening. Do take care.'

My own doctor wasn't on duty at the surgery when I arrived but another female doctor in the practice saw me. I told her what had happened.

'You poor thing.' She looked at me sympathetically.

'What really worries me is that I'm incontinent.'

'It doesn't sound like it. Let's just examine you.'

The pain was still so sharp that I could show her exactly where it was.

'Your colon has gone into spasm. What with that, the pressure in the aircraft and the strong laxative in the tablets you were given I'm not really surprised what happened. You're not incontinent.'

'A *laxative*? I didn't know that. I should have been told.'

I went home and ran a hot bath. It felt safe to hide in the bathroom and as I soaked in the water the pain in my stomach eased away. I was angry that I hadn't been told what was in the tablets. I should have asked for the exact details. How stupid of me! It also struck me that without MS, the thought of being incontinent wouldn't have crossed my mind.

I was afraid, though. For one thing, my manager had seen me in a complete mess for the first time. And what would the crew think if this story went round the airline? They all knew by now that I had MS, but I'd always looked perfectly all right. Would this episode change their attitude towards me?

I climbed out of the bath, wrapped myself in a towelling robe, and went downstairs. Just then, Julie came walking in.

'Hi, Carole. How was your day?'

'It was a *nightmare.*' I started to laugh. 'I should have stayed at home in bed. Do you want to hear about it before you eat or after?'

I had a few days off work but I had to brave going back sometime. The crew on the Bilbao flight had been upset by seeing me so ill. I felt it was my task to make a joke out of it.

'Are you feeling better?' one of the crew asked on my first day back.

'Well, what can I say? Shit happens! Now I've proved it.' Everyone laughed – and then the stories started to come out.

There's one thing about being caught short in a public place – loads of people who don't have MS have had similar experiences. I got to hear them all. The point is, not everything boils down to MS – but what an embarrassing way to make my point!

The summer of 1995 was slipping away and, after the frenzy of my charity event, things had gone flat. So it seemed logical to do another one. I decided I'd organize a champagne reception this time around. I rarely drink, but if I do I like it to be champagne. I went back on the trail for sponsors.

I chose Stringfellows club as the venue again as it had been so successful the last time, and then an invitation to Peter Stringfellow's birthday party landed on my doormat. The afternoon of the party the MS Society rang.

'Carole, Channel Four have rung. They want to interview you for a documentary.' David Harrison, the society's press officer, sounded pleased.

'*Me.* Whatever for?'

'It's a programme about taking responsibility for your own health.'

'If it's positive and I can be myself, I'd be interested.' I put the phone down.

A little while later a Channel Four researcher rang and interviewed me for an hour.

'Carole, you sound exactly what we're after. Can we come and see you tomorrow, say nine o'clock, for a proper interview?'

'Do you mean nine in the morning? I'll be at a party tonight so I might feel a bit rough. I'm just warning you.'

'What do you mean? You still go out and party?'

'Of course I do. See you tomorrow.'

By the time I reached Stringfellows I felt like celebrating. I was excited at the thought of the documentary. And after I'd spoken to Channel Four, the champagne company Piper Heidsieck had agreed to sponsor my champagne reception. What a day! I joined a group of friends and started on the Buck's Fizz as I was telling them all about it.

Looking round the packed club, I saw someone I thought I knew and was just about to wave at him when a member of the club's staff came over for a chat.

'Who's that guy standing over there? He looks so familiar,' I said.

'That's Sid Owen. You know, he plays Ricky in *EastEnders*.'

'Thank goodness I didn't make a prat of myself. I thought it was somebody I knew.'

'I'll introduce you to him. Come on.'

We walked over to him and after the introductions, she left us. I didn't want to waste his time, so waded straight in.

'I don't want to bother you now, but I do charity events for multiple sclerosis.'

'Why MS?' he asked.

'Because I've got it.' He looked at me more closely.

'No way!'

'Yes. I wondered, would you come along to my next event?'

'Yes, no problem. Is that what you do for a living?'

'No. I'm a British Airways stewardess.'

He laughed. 'Let's do a deal. You get me some cheap flights, and I'll get you some celebrities!'

We swapped phone numbers and chatted a bit more, then I made my way outside, breathed in the sharp night air and decided it was time to go home. I loved champagne but it didn't love me!

The next morning the assistant producer of the documentary came to my house. She told me I'd have a 12-minute slot on a programme called *The Pulse*. They wanted to start filming at the beginning of November. Just then my phone rang.

'Hi, Carole. It's Sid here. We met last night.'

'Hi, how are you doing?'

'I just wanted you to know that I meant what I said last night.'

'Oh that's great. Thanks very much for ringing. Speak to you soon.'

I was glad he'd rung; I had already lost his phone number! Sid and I have been friends ever since.

The documentary's director, Hugh Whitworth, met me a few days later so that I could take him around the locations he wanted to film. Two weeks later filming began. As the crew trooped in to the house, with lights, cameras and tons of equipment, I suddenly felt very nervous. This is television! That means lots of people will see it. It dawned on me what I had let myself in for.

'OK, Carole. We'll warm you up slowly. Let's have you talking on the phone, sitting just over here.' He pointed to the dining table.

'Who am I talking to?'

'Well, I'll phone you and you can make it up as we go along.'

I entered the weird world of filming, and loved it. The crew liked me, for a very simple reason. I was so nervous that I kept asking for cigarette breaks. They were all smokers so it gave them a chance to smoke, too. We filmed and filmed, at home, on my own, with friends, at Stringfellows. We had started at 8.30 in the morning and I crawled into bed at 4.30 the next morning. All that was left to do were the shots of me in uniform at Heathrow and they were scheduled for the next week.

Then I fell ill. It was only a flu bug, but it floored me. I rang Ricky from The Untouchables to ask if he'd drive me to the doctor's surgery. He lived nearby now with his girlfriend, Tracy Coleman, a model and Page Three girl. When they arrived, she had come straight from a photo shoot and was looking her most glamorous. The journey to the surgery was agonizing; every jolt in the car, or going over speed bumps in the road, sent pain through all my joints. The three of us walked into the waiting-room. Four young men sitting in one corner looked up and their jaws dropped as they realized who the stunning blonde about to sit next to them was. I sat looking like death warmed up until my name was called.

When we arrived back at my house, Tracy went into the kitchen to make us all a coffee.

'Carole, you're almost out of milk,' she said. 'Shall we go and do your shopping for you?' She and Ricky stocked up my fridge as I sat and contemplated another three weeks at home.

I went back to work with a cameraman hanging out of my car window. The film crew had arrived early and asked me to put on my make-up and my hat standing in front of the living-room mirror. The idea that any stewardess would wear her hat on the way to work was ridiculous but I understood that it made good TV. The scene took ages; trying to put on blusher in front of a film crew made me nervous and every time I looked into the mirror I laughed. Then I had a fit of the giggles and we had to stop filming for a while until I was calm again. All the time, people walking past my house were staring in through the door and windows.

I was very self-conscious during the filming at Heathrow. I had persuaded my friend Denise Rothwell to be with me in some of the scenes and she helped enormously. I didn't feel so conspicuous with two of us in uniform in front of the cameras. We did exactly as we were told, going up and down escalators, checking into work, chatting 'naturally' – even though the arc lights were blinding us both.

I had to gatecrash a briefing, which was embarrassing enough, but then the director asked me to stand at an aircraft door to be filmed welcoming passengers on board. I had no idea where they were going so just smiled, saying: 'Good morning. I hope you enjoy your flight,' until the cameramen had what they needed.

Friends kept coming over to say hello – then ran a mile when they saw the cameras. Everywhere we went all day there was a flurry of activity. The camera crew, the local newspapers, the British Airways newspaper. I was never alone. The last scene of the day was a reflexology session with Denise. It was good to be away from the airport and as she quietly described what she was doing to my feet I could feel myself relaxing. I was shattered.

Despite the exhaustion, I was sorry to see the crew go when filming ended. I'd been so nervous when I first met them and now it seemed odd driving home on my own. In fact, I missed them. I never lived down my moment of fame at work, though.

One evening just before Christmas Julie and I sat chatting in the living-room of our house. 'Carole, do you think you would have done your charity event and everything else if you'd still been with Craig?'

'I don't know.' I thought for a while. 'I think Craig and I had to end our relationship for me to be free to do all these things.'

'Do you still think about him? You never mention him.'

'I think Craig leaving me was the best thing he could have done. He and Tracy did me a big favour!' Julie smiled.

'I think you're right.'

After Christmas I had a phone call from the tenants who were renting my old flat to say they were moving out. Two days later, our landlord rang us to say he wanted to sell the house. Julie and I would have to leave within three months. We sat down to discuss what to do next.

'Carole, I've decided that now's the time to move in with Mark.'

Julie and her boyfriend had been thinking about this for a while and it seemed right. But what would I do?

'Why don't you move back into your old flat?' Julie suggested. The idea hadn't crossed my mind. Sara from the beauty salon I attended needed somewhere to live and said she would rent my spare bedroom. As the idea grew on me I decided to refurnish and redecorate the flat. I didn't want to live with the ghosts of my time there with Craig.

The timing was dreadful. I had so much to do again and the last thing I'd expected was to move house at the start of 1996. Channel Four had already sent me some copies of the documentary on video but I put them away in a cupboard. I'm very self-critical and knew I would feel happier watching it for the first time with my friends around me when it was screened. Things didn't work out like that.

The documentary was due to be shown on TV at 8 p.m. on 2 February. BBC Radio Four rang and asked me to appear on a health and disabilities programme, *Does He Take Sugar*? But, just like the night of my charity event the previous year, they wanted me on the night of the screening and their programme began at 8.30 p.m. I agreed, if I could watch the documentary at BBC Broadcasting House.

When I arrived I spotted Peter Cardy, the MS Society chief executive, standing in reception. I had seen pictures of him but we had never met. He recognized me, too.

'I've seen your programme, Carole,' he said shaking my hand. 'I think you'll be pleased with it.'

We headed for a small room with a TV. It was difficult getting tuned to Channel Four in the BBC headquarters and for a moment we thought we'd miss the beginning but then it started.

'That hair's got to go. I look like Miss Piggy!' I burst out as I saw my face on the TV screen for the first time. Peter laughed but then we fell silent and listened.

As I heard myself talking about my illness the tears started streaming down my face. It had been so hectic during the filming that I had hardly noticed what I was saying. It was the first time I had spoken with such honesty and it made me feel very emotional. The director had ended the documentary with me saying: 'I've got MS, but it hasn't got me – at least, not yet.' As the credits rolled I tried to dry my eyes. I shouldn't have agreed to do this. I needed my friends to be with me.

I felt a wreck as we made our way to the recording studio. I'd started the week with a night-stop in Istanbul and that morning I'd had a 4 a.m. alarm call. I really wasn't at my best. But everything went smoothly. The interviewer showed an interest in alternative therapies so I could talk about the things I knew. Peter Cardy backed me up when I suggested it was best to be open-minded.

'We haven't any guarantees, but people should use whatever suits them,' he said.

I was glad that I'd kept to my resolution to keep myself up-to-date about MS. It meant I could avoid the panic I'd felt in my first radio interviews and that helped me to relax, too. I was getting better at going public!

'They tell me you're organizing another event,' Peter said as we strolled to the front door of Broadcasting House. 'Have you set a date for it?'

'Yes, 23 April. Will you be there?'

'Let's meet for lunch and have a chat. I'll bring along David Harrison from the press office, too. How about that?'

'I'd love to. Nice meeting you, Peter. Bye.'

I made my way straight to my friend Melanie's house where I knew she and her sister, Maxine, were waiting for me. All the way there my mobile phone was ringing. The impact of the TV programme really hit me; most of my family and friends had heard me talking from my heart about MS for the first time and they were a bit emotional about it. Perhaps it had made it real for them. Even my dad rang to say he and his wife had been crying. But sitting in the car, speaking into my mobile, I felt completely calm.

I arrived at Melanie's and as she opened the door, Maxine came walking up the hallway.

'We're so proud of you,' Maxine said as Melanie closed the front door. I stood in the hall and burst into tears. It was really all too much for me.

The next day, Julie and I sat at home and watched the programme again. We were both crying by the end. I had sent a copy of the video of the programme to Mum in Australia and she had left a message on my answer phone. She'd been struggling not to cry, too. I hadn't realized that putting my illness into words would release so much emotion, not just for me but also for the people close to me. Again, my phone didn't stop ringing all day – friends, people from work, and then David Harrison from the MS Society.

'Hello, Carole. Congratulations on last night's programme.'

'Thanks, David. I can't see it yet without bursting into tears.'

'Look, there's a conference coming up in London. About 200 neurologists and doctors. We thought we'd show your video. Would that be OK with you?'

'Of course, you don't need to ask.'

'Yes, but we'd like you there, to give a speech. Could you manage that without crying?' He laughed down the phone.

'I can't speak in front of all those people!'

'Well done, Carole. I knew you'd say yes.'

I felt dreadful when I walked into the Copthorne Hotel in Kensington. Acres of round dining tables and not one face that I recognized. I had learnt that I preferred doing my public appearances on my own. Perhaps I felt better about talking to strangers. I could keep myself detached if there was nobody close to me in the audience. And in the early days, it had never crossed my mind to ask for permission for a friend to come with me. Then David Harrison came up to me.

'Are you all right, Carole? By the way, at the end of your speech, would you announce dinner?'

'At least I'm speaking before the meal, then,' I said, laughing. I sat down feeling lost. Then I spotted MS Society chief executive Peter Cardy's bearded and friendly face and smiled and waved.

Everyone settled into their seats and my video came up on a cinema-sized screen at one end of the room. When it came to the scene of Denise giving me reflexology, my feet filled the screen, ten feet high, two feet wide. I looked down at the tablecloth, desperately trying not to laugh. As the video ended, I had to get up and walk onto the stage to the microphone. As I got there, a blinding spotlight was put on me. This is my idea of hell, I kept thinking. Then I looked up and realized that because of the lighting I couldn't see the audience. It was a blessing in disguise.

I had decided not to write a speech but to talk about my experience of multiple sclerosis. I didn't make it too personal, although I couldn't resist a plug for my next charity event. I ended by saying: 'On behalf of all of us, I would like to thank all of you for your hard work in research. Let's hope we're one step closer to finding a cure for multiple sclerosis. Good luck and bon appetit!'

I was still shaking half an hour later and the meal passed in a blur. To be honest, I was out of my league – surrounded by professors and other researchers. We all had an interest in multiple sclerosis but from very different perspectives. However, I sold 100 tickets for my event, mainly to staff from London's Institute of Neurology, and I had one conversation with a researcher I shall never forget.

'Carole? Hello, I'm working in research into MS and just wanted to say how nice it is to meet you.'

'Thank you. I'm glad I came.'

'Researchers aren't like doctors and neurologists, we rarely meet someone who actually has MS. We're stuck in the lab all week.'

'I hadn't thought of it like that.'

He made me think. For that reason alone it had been worth an attack of the nerves. At least I'd been able to thank them all which is probably why I agreed to go through it all again a few weeks later in the even grander setting of London's Science Museum. The audience that time was the MS Federation, a worldwide organization. The video was shown again and watching peoples' reactions to it I began to get the seed of a very exciting idea.

I was struggling to keep up day-to-day. I was organizing my second event and redecorating my flat. Flying was taking more and more out of me, too. Anyone, MS or not, would feel stressed.

In fact, I had been so busy that my friend Maxine had rung twice to organize an evening together and I'd had to put her off. The first time, she'd had a cold. I was learning to avoid cold and flu bugs as much as I could so I had stayed away. The second time I was just too tired to go out and had cancelled. So we arranged a third date to meet. I had been at work that day and felt exhausted. I knew Maxine would understand so I rang her at home.

'Hi, Maxine. I'm really sorry but I'm going to cancel again. I feel worn out. I'm not up to a night out.'

'Oh, no. Why don't you come over and stay the night?'

'No, I really don't feel like it.'

'Oh. go on, Carole. It's ages since I've seen you.'

'Sorry, Max. I just can't.' Maxine put the phone down.

I was really upset; she was the last friend I would have expected to do that. I waited for about half-an-hour, then rang her back.

'Are you angry with me, Max?'

'Well, you have let me down three times now.'

'I know and I'm sorry. You understand though, don't you? I've just been so tired lately. It's not that I don't want to see you.'

'I do understand. But I have problems, too, and I need to see you. I can't come to you because Paul's working late and he's got the car.'

'I know, and I want to be there for you. But I just can't tonight.'

'I don't want to put more pressure on you, Carole, you know that.'

'I know, Max. I feel like I haven't seen you for ages.'

'I'll tell you what. How about we stay in and I'll cook you dinner. You can stay the night. No pressure!'

'God, I haven't even thought about dinner. I haven't had time to do any shopping. That's a great idea.'

It made me think. My friends needed me as much as I needed them and it was hard if they felt they needed to tiptoe around me because of my MS. I was glad Maxine had shown me how she felt. It made me aware I had to plan my meetings with friends more carefully. If they were making allowances for me, I'd have to make sure I had time for them, too.

I had a night-stop in Copenhagen a week before Julie and I were due to move out of our house. The flight home meant yet another 4 a.m. alarm call and later, as I was driving home through London, my mobile phone flashed with a string of messages. I had so much to do before I could go to bed but all I wanted was to rest.

I dropped off to sleep at about 10 that night. Just as my body began to relax I suddenly felt an electric current run from the top of my head to my feet. That's the only way I can describe it. I couldn't open my mouth to speak. My arms and legs were paralyzed, too. If I'd been sleeping with anyone I wouldn't have been able to wake them up for help. None of the usual messages were getting through to my brain. It was as though my body didn't belong to me. But after about a minute it stopped. I sat up in bed slowly, terrified. What was it? What if that happened again but kept on and on? Was it the MS?

The next morning I phoned the neurologist at the Atkinson Morley Hospital. 'What is going on?' I asked after I'd described what had happened.

'Well, you'd been rushing around all day and when your body relaxed you could have had a relapse.'

'It only lasted about a minute.'

'Relapses can last just minutes.'

'I didn't know that.'

'Or it could have been night-time paralysis. That can happen to anybody. But I can't really tell you what it was.'

I saw this as a warning sign, flashing on and off in huge letters and bright colours. PUT YOUR HEALTH FIRST! But what could I do? I had to move house, I had to keep working to pay the bills and my event was only weeks away. For the first time in ages I wished I wasn't single. If only I had someone to share the responsibilities and take some of the pressure off me. From that day on, I was very concerned about what might happen if I didn't slow down. But I had no choice.

Julie and I moved out a few days later. She had been a very supportive and understanding flatmate and, although we would remain best friends, I was going to miss her. But I was glad I wouldn't be alone in my flat and that Sara would be around. I'd had some frightening symptoms in the last few months and having Julie in the house had taken some of the fear away. Just as I was learning to go public I was discovering that the most important thing for me is to have someone to go home to.

15. Turbulence

I looked into the mirror and saw a new me. My second charity event was beginning in a few hours' time. I'd already had a body massage and facial, manicure and pedicure at the beauty salon run by Sofie and my flatmate Sara. Now our hairdresser friend Debbie had cut off my hair. I had hated my old style since I saw myself in the TV documentary. The day's pampering had been a surprise treat.

'Carole, you were exhausted after your last event,' Sara had said to me in my flat the night before. 'This time around, you must enjoy it. No arguments; you're to spend the day at our salon.'

She was right. I needed to be told to relax. The haircut was a bonus. I loved it! Once I'd put on my new pink jacket and black trousers I felt ready for anything, which was just as well because I arrived at Stringfellows club and walked into a nightmare. Everything seemed to be going wrong.

The girl on the door couldn't make the till accept the £12 cost of an entrance ticket. Either £10 or £20 was fine, but nothing in-between. I was trying to figure that out when another member of staff came up to me.

'There are two coaches from British Airways outside. Where shall I tell them to park?'

I had no idea, although I felt for the people in the coaches, being kept waiting with the engines running outside. 'Wherever they would normally park,' I answered, turning away before the man asking had time to question me further.

Everything sorted itself out and soon I was sitting at a table in the middle of the club. This time I wanted people to find me rather than have to run around after them. I was learning!

One man, Ivan Jackson, had phoned me weeks earlier to ask about wheelchair access. I'd told him: 'Don't worry, whatever happens we'll figure something out.' Now here he was, much younger than I'd expected, asking me for the first dance.

I was whisked onto the dance floor and Ivan made that chair dance, there's no other word for it. I was impressed. Here was someone who wanted to have a good time and he knew how to do it, too.

The club filled quickly and soon 700 people had come through the door. As the champagne began to flow Sid Owen from *EastEnders*, true to his word, arrived with lots of the boys from the soap's cast – Paul Nichols, who played Joe, Dean Gaffney (Robbie), Steve McFadden, Phil in the soap, and Mark Homer, or Tony as fans know him. The actress Barbara Windsor arrived later to keep the boys under control. My friend Ricky's girlfriend, Tracy Coleman, made her first public appearance that evening, too, after featuring as a Page Three girl.

'Carole, you will stand next to me, won't you?' she said when I asked her if she would announce a raffle prize on stage.

'Of course I will, Tracy. Don't worry. You'll be fine.' I sounded like an old hand and I was enjoying myself. I didn't have to perform on stage like I had last time and I could sit at my table and relax when I wanted. Then a woman about the same age as me came over.

'Carole, I just wanted to tell you that I saw your documentary and found it really inspiring.' She held my hand as I stood up and I realized how tiny she was. I towered over her.

'Thank you. Are you enjoying yourself?'

'I'm having a lovely time.'

I took a deep breath to ask the obvious question.

'You said you enjoyed the documentary. Do you have MS?'

'Yes,' she said. 'My situation is a bit more complicated, though. I've been diagnosed with cancer, too.'

I didn't know what to say. Why on earth would anyone be handed such a bad deal in life? It didn't make sense. We chatted for ages and she told me that she had only a few months to live. I thought about her for the rest of the evening. How could I have inspired *her* when she was managing to face life against the cruellest of odds?

I had asked this time not to be told how much money we had raised, although everyone knew it was my dream to make £10,000. Just as I climbed the steps to the stage to oversee the raffle a Piper Heidsieck champagne company representative leaned over to me.

'I hope you won't be disappointed. We didn't reach your goal.'

'Oh well, we've all had a good time. Never mind,' I said. I meant it, too. We'd had fun and everything had gone smoothly after the first hiccups.

Neil Fox was the DJ on stage again, along with loads of celebrities who were presenting raffle prizes. Then Neil announced at the microphone: 'Carole's dream tonight is to raise £10,000.'

I wanted the stage to swallow me up. Oh no, nobody's told him we didn't make it.

'So,' Neil continued, 'I'll just hold up this cheque for you all to see.'

He looked straight at me and began to unroll a huge presentation cheque. I saw the letter 'T', then 'E' and 'N'. TEN! We had hit our target. They'd been winding me up. Ten thousand pounds! I burst into tears, of course. What else would I do? My dream had come true. Neil hugged me. Then Sid Owen took the microphone and turned to me.

'My friend Mem has written this song and we're going to sing it for Carole.'

Everyone applauded and I didn't know where to look as Mem and Sid started to sing to me.

The rest of the evening passed like a dream, I felt so happy. I had time to chat with people and I didn't feel panicky. I looked back and realized I had taken on far too much with my first event.

I was the last to leave the club again and went home with the presentation cheque under my arm. Back at my flat I unrolled it, spread it across my sofa and sat staring at it until dawn. Half the money would go towards research into multiple sclerosis and the other half would put a new roof on a holiday home for the disabled. That reality was what made me feel so fulfilled. The cheque was just money but it represented real help for real people and it was the most thrilling thing I could do. There was only one person I wanted to share my feelings with. At 5 a.m. I picked up the phone to ring my mum in Australia.

'Mum, guess what! We raised £10,000!'

'Well done. That's wonderful. I wish I could have been there.'

'I can't believe it.'

'You sound tired, darling.'

'I am, I'm exhausted. But I'm too excited to sleep.'

A few weeks later, in June, 1996, I was sitting with Marci King at her London home. My friend Julie had been nanny to Marci's son before she went into teaching and Marci had known me since I was 17.

'When did you last have a proper holiday?' she asked me out of the blue. I couldn't remember.

'Take our villa, Carole, and have a good rest. Do you promise?'

It was too good an offer to turn down. A week in the Algarve with nothing to do but sit by the pool.

'I'd love that, Marci. Thanks.'

I came home from Portugal tanned, relaxed and looking forward to work. It was a great summer. I felt well and confident.

My manager at BA, Maggie, had been encouraging me gently to think of jobs that didn't involve flying.

'I'm just pointing out,' she said to me in her office one day, 'that if for any reason you can't fly you should have something to fall back on. Perhaps a qualification that will make it possible to work somewhere else within BA?'

'But I love flying. I don't want to do anything else.'

I couldn't imagine a day when I would have to give up my job. At the same time, I knew that what Maggie was saying was sensible. So when I heard about a public relations and marketing course at a college in Kensington, I made some inquiries. Classes were every Saturday so I could manage that. But you needed a degree or 'A' Levels to take part. I went to see the college principal.

'I've organized two big charity events and been interviewed on radio and in the press,' I argued. 'Surely that's worth more than an 'A'

Level?' I put my folder of press cuttings on his desk. He looked through it slowly.

'You're right. You're in,' he said and smiled at me. Maggie was delighted.

'I think you'd be good in this field, Carole. It doesn't mean you have to give up flying now, but it gives you more options if you feel differently in the future.'

I was really excited at being a student. I had rebelled when I was 14 and living in Banff in Scotland. I had hated school and it was no secret that I considered the day I had left Inverurie Academy as one of the happiest of my life. Now I had a second chance. It was a lot of work to take on while I was flying full-time, but for the first few weeks I really enjoyed myself. Then I was told I needed to have my wisdom teeth removed.

It's a common operation so I was surprised when the consultant at St George's Hospital in Tooting advised me not to have a general anaesthetic.

'It can trigger a relapse in MS,' he said. 'It would be better to have a milder local anaesthetic.'

'No way! I'm petrified of dentists. I can't have the operation if I can see what you're doing. I can't go through with it unless I can have a proper anaesthetic,' I told him.

So I was booked in at the hospital for three days and put in a room on my own. I was due to be operated on the next morning and the rest of the evening stretched ahead. I was bored.

'Can I leave the hospital for a meal when my sister arrives?' I asked the nursing sister on duty.

'No, you mustn't leave the building, I'm afraid.'

'Can I at least go downstairs to the restaurant?'

'OK. But be back here by 9 p.m. You need to rest before the op.'

When Hazel and her husband Paul arrived the three of us nipped out for a meal in an Indian restaurant down the road. How would anyone know as long as I was back on the ward in time?

By the next morning I was very nervous. The warning of a possible relapse was playing on my mind. What if I couldn't walk when I come round? What if I had a bad relapse that lasted for months?

I woke up in the recovery room with my mouth packed with cotton wool and an oxygen mask strapped onto my face. I felt panicky and ripped the mask off. Can I walk? Can I walk? I needed to know. I had to lie still for an hour, surrounded by other patients who were all sleeping soundly. Eventually I was wheeled back up to my room.

Once I was alone I tried lifting each of my limbs in turn. My legs wouldn't move and the panic was rising. Calm down, calm down, I kept saying to myself. It took me two hours to be able to sit up in bed. Through the window of my room I could see another woman in the main ward who'd had the same op as me. She was still asleep. My fear of a relapse must have been so strong that it had forced me awake more quickly.

My whole body felt heavy but I swung my legs over the side of the bed and sat still, willing myself to stand up. I had to know whether I was all right. I got onto my feet feeling shaky and sick. I walked a few steps across my room, then through the door and out into the corridor. I was half way down, guiding myself with one hand leaning on the wall, when a doctor called out.

'What on earth are you doing?'

I turned around and looked at him.

'I had to know whether I could walk,' I said. 'I'm sorry. It's all I could think about.' He walked towards me.

'Would you go back to bed now? You must rest.'

I lay in my bed, relieved that my legs were working. When the specialist came to see me later in the afternoon he advised that I should stay in hospital for another few days.

'I really would like to go home,' I pleaded.

'Is there anyone at home to be with you?'

'Yes,' I lied, knowing that my flatmate Sara wouldn't be there for hours.

The other wisdom teeth patient came into my room for a chat. I discovered that she lived round the corner from me. When her husband came to pick her up, I discharged myself and they gave me a lift home.

I felt fine; I was on painkillers so my face wasn't hurting and after a long bath I was just relieved that I'd managed to have a general anaesthetic with no side-effects. Later in the evening I began to have nose-bleeds. I rang the hospital.

'Don't worry. That's quite common. It's a reaction to all the tubes we use during the operation. They'll go away,' I was told.

The next day I had the most dreadful pains in my head. Sara stayed with me all day, massaging my head and forehead. But each time she stopped, the pain came back. When I woke up the next morning and lifted my head the most awful pain hit me. I remembered the day of my lumbar puncture in Rio before I was first diagnosed with MS. I cried and cried.

This time Sara took me back to the hospital. The specialist checked me over and said: 'It's nothing to do with the operation you've had. I think you should see your neurologist.'

We climbed back into the car and Sara drove me to the Atkinson Morley Hospital. I was examined again, this time by the neurologist.

'Well, you're not having a relapse, Carole. It's just a reaction to the operation. You must rest. Your body has had a shock.'

I needed two weeks off work to recover. I had been an idiot. I should have kept still and quiet after the operation, but fear had forced me onto my feet. And I should have stayed in hospital instead of discharging myself. I would never do that again. By the time I went back to work I had admitted the truth: I had brought a lot of the pain on myself.

I tried to use night-stops from then on as an opportunity to study for my course. Crew can be very persuasive, though, and often I'd give in and spend the evening with them instead. Eventually I hit on the idea of taking none of my ordinary clothes with me. I had only a change of uniform. We weren't allowed to go out on the town in uniform – not that I'd want to – so I had no choice but to stay in my hotel room and work. It wasn't much fun, but it was the only way I could catch up and do myself justice. It just seemed to be such a busy time.

On 14 October, 1996, I made my only appearance on live TV. The date is engraved on my heart as the worst experience in my quest to make people aware of MS. Where should I begin?

I arrived at the Talk TV studios in Southwark, London, and met Shirley Meadows. She was the main reason I had agreed to go on the Second Opinion health programme. Shirley has a progressive form of MS and I have always been keen that all types of MS should be discussed. We got chatting as I wheeled her into the studio and joked that we were as nervous as one another.

It soon became clear that the team making the programme hadn't expected a wheelchair user. One of the presenters said: 'Where are we going to put the wheelchair, where shall we put Shirley?'

'You don't want to be on the settee, do you Shirley?' a producer asked.

'No, I don't,' Shirley told him.

I was outraged at the lack of sensitivity. Eventually, I had acres of sofa to myself and Shirley was stuck at the end, almost out of camera shot. 'Can you tell us what we'll have to do?' I spotted a researcher standing near one of the five cameras and caught her eye.

'Oh, just talk about MS,' she replied. Great help! I raised my eyebrows at Shirley as she smiled and shook her head.

The programme began and I was so nervous I wanted to be sick. I managed to speak and Shirley kept calm, too. Inside, we were both shaking. That turned to panic when the presenters announced there was a phone-in. I was petrified that someone would ask a question I couldn't answer. But the first caller was cut off and none of them had questions. They just wanted to tell their stories. The expert, on videophone, had trouble with his sound and at one point there was an uncomfortable silence. We all looked at one another; it lasted five seconds and felt like five minutes. As the whole thing disintegrated I could almost see the funny side of things.

As soon as the programme ended, I wheeled Shirley out onto the landing. It was a 'No Smoking' building, but we found ourselves a hideaway and had a cigarette.

'That was pathetic!'

'Do you think it was worth it?' Shirley asked.

I suppose it was if the programme helped one person with MS. I've only shown the tape to three people; it makes me cringe. I know if I ever have to do live TV again, I shall be a nervous wreck. At least it couldn't be worse.

A few days later I went down with flu. I had just recovered and was on a flight to Prague when the internal phone at the back of the plane rang.

'Carole, check out the passenger sitting in 23C.' It was the stewardess working at the front of the plane. 'It's an aisle seat. He's absolutely gorgeous!'

On my way down the aisle I glanced at the man sitting in 23C. She was right. He had jet black hair, piercing blue eyes and the biggest smile, which he beamed at me as I walked past.

'He's a bit of all right!' I said when I got back to the galley. We all calmed down and got on with our work, then the aircraft hit bad turbulence.

'Could all cabin crew please be seated and put on seat belts,' the pilot's voice came through on our phone. As we sat down another stewardess said to me: '23C is interested in you, Carole. Give him your number.'

'No way. I never have before with a passenger and I'm not starting now,' I replied, laughing. She started to scribble on a piece of paper.

'I'm giving him this unless you make the first move,' she said, handing me the paper. I read what was on it.

'Roses are red, violets are blue, turbulence is great, and so are you. Carole.'

'Speak to him or I'll give him this and tell him which hotel we're staying at,' she said, grinning. We were like schoolgirls!

I knew I wouldn't speak to Mr 23C so when we'd passed through the turbulence and were out clearing the meal trays I was shocked to hear the stewardess say to him: 'This is from Carole.' The piece of paper was handed to him. I blushed bright red, ducked to hide behind the trolley and knocked everything off the top. Bottles, glasses, napkins, all went flying down the aisle.

Five minutes later my cupid stewardess came into the galley.

'23C asked me to give you this,' she said. It was his business card with a note: 'Meet me in the hotel lobby at 8 p.m., Stefan.'

'Oh great,' I said after reading it. 'Just when I don't have a change of clothes with me.'

The crew dressed me that evening; one lent me a black crocheted jumper (I had only a white bra with me, so it didn't look very sophisticated); another gave me her black leggings which had thick white stripes down each leg; and to complete the look someone else gave me her black boots – she'd walked her dogs in them that morning and they left a trail of dried mud.

'I can't go out looking like this!' I wailed as the crew stood around assuring me that I looked fine.

'Carole, he's in the lobby.' One of the stewardesses had spotted him downstairs, already waiting.

'Oh well, here goes,' I said and went down in the lift not quite believing what I had let myself in for.

I strode over to Stefan and he gave me his beaming smile.

'I have two things to say before we go anywhere, Stefan,' I said.

'Sure, go ahead.'

'Firstly, I didn't write that poem you were given on the plane. Secondly, these are not my clothes.'

'No problem. Now, shall we have some cocktails?' He had a German accent. I hadn't really thought where he would be from.

He took me to a trendy cocktail bar in the city centre. We entered at street level but had to go down a flight of stairs to reach the bar. It struck me how beautifully dressed everyone was. I looked down and noticed that I'd left bits of dried mud on each step. There was probably more of it in his car! This wasn't a good start.

Stefan turned out to be charming, funny and very attentive. He didn't take his eyes off me and we spent most of the evening laughing. I told him that I had MS and handed him a card which I always carry in case of an emergency. '*I have MS. It is not infectious. Please can you help?*' It's written in French, Spanish, Italian and German.

'I just want to make sure you really understand what I'm saying.' I looked at him.

'I do understand. A friend of mine has multiple sclerosis.'

That was it. As the evening went on it crossed my mind that he was perhaps a bit too perfect. But I hadn't been on a proper date for ages so I was probably a bit rusty.

'When are you coming back to Prague?' he asked as he delivered me back at the hotel.

'I've no idea, it depends on my roster,' I said.

'I'll give you a call, Carole.' He gave me a kiss on the cheek and left.

He did call, the next day, which impressed me. When I arrived back at Heathrow I was even more surprised that I was rostered to return to Prague the next month.

I went down with the flu a second time and realized – yet again – that I was doing too much. Working full-time and going to college was wearing me out. My college course had proved to me that I couldn't bear the thought of not flying. I knew I had to broaden my options, but not just yet.

One Saturday at college I met up with my friend Denise for lunch in Kensington. As stewardesses we went months without seeing one another and had set this date to make sure we could catch up with each other's news. As she made her way to my table in the restaurant I was struck by her immaculate good taste. She was wearing a simple black jumper and black trousers, her long black hair loose over her shoulders and her hallmark red lipstick applied perfectly, as ever. She was laden down with carrier bags.

'You look stunning as usual, Denise,' I said laughing as she came over to my table. 'How do you do it?' We gave each other a hug.

'I hear you've been poorly, Carole.' She hadn't even sat down. I couldn't keep anything from Denise.

'I think my immune system's low at the moment.'

She started to tell me off. 'Don't overdo it. Make time for yourself. You must.'

'Yes, but what am I supposed to do? I still need to pay the bills. It's all down to me.'

'Maybe this course will help you to go in another direction. You're happiest doing your charity events, aren't you?'

'I don't think PR and marketing are right for me. I'm already doing what I love. I want to keep being a stewardess.'

'There's more to life than just flying, you know.'

I told Denise my Prague story. We both laughed so loudly that people at other tables turned round to see what was happening.

On my next visit to Prague, just before Christmas, Stefan called to say he wanted to surprise me. This time I took my own clothes to change into. When he arrived at the hotel to pick me up, I took one look at him and thought: 'God, I don't remember him being *that* gorgeous!'

He drove me to an old building in the city centre with huge oak doors. As he opened them I peeked inside to see a stone staircase curving up with two candles glowing on each step. I suddenly felt uneasy.

'Where are you taking me?'

'Trust me, Carole. Keep going.'

Oh no, what if this is his apartment? Then two doors at the top of the staircase opened and there was the most breathtakingly romantic restaurant I had ever seen. A Christmas tree twinkled in the middle of the floor, there were candles on each table, and through the window I could see Prague Palace. We had a fabulous meal and Stefan was fun. I liked the fact that in such posh surroundings he was prepared to be silly. We flicked bread crumbs at each other, and at one point he threw his napkin and it landed on my head. He took me back to my hotel and we said goodnight.

'What happened, Carole? Come on, tell us.' Some of my crew were in the hotel lounge, agog for details.

'Nothing. We had a really good time and he's good company. But my gut feeling keeps telling me that nobody's *that* perfect.'

My stepfather Ivan paid for my sister and me to fly to Australia for Christmas, along with his daughters who flew across Australia to Perth from their home in Victoria. He wanted all of his family together in the new house he and my mum had moved into in Canning Vale. For the first time, we could have a room each – and at last they had a swimming pool. I was looking forward to Australia; I felt I had been ill on and off since my wisdom teeth operation and I always heal in Perth.

But on Christmas Eve morning I woke up with a swollen throat, barely able to swallow, and felt dreadful. Oh not again. I just wanted to be well!

I walked into the kitchen where Mum was up to her elbows in preparations for the next day. She looked at me and knew immediately that something was wrong.

'I don't feel well,' I said and started to cry. She stopped everything and took me to her doctor.

'Carole Mackie?' The receptionist called my name and Mum and I both stood up. We walked into the surgery.

'Now what seems to be the problem?' the doctor asked, looking at me. I turned and looked at my mum as she started telling him – I let her, too! We all three laughed as we realized what had happened. I was a little girl again, with mummy taking me to the doctor's.

I was put on antibiotics and Christmas came and went. I didn't feel well but during the next week my tongue became sore. I stuck it out for mum to take a look.

'Oh yuk! It's white,' she said. The antibiotics had caused a reaction. How attractive! Whatever was going to strike next?

When I went back to work I had yet another night-stop in Prague. Stefan and I had a wonderful date; a gorgeous meal and a snowball fight outside the restaurant as the evening ended. He was as charming as ever.

The next morning I got onto the crew bus for the trip to the airport. As I sat down I shouted out: 'Wow! Heated seats. That's what I call luxury.'

Other crew looked at me.

'Mine's not heated,' they each started to say.

'Come and try mine.' I stood up to let a steward have a go.

'That's not hot, Carole,' he said.

My back was burning. It had gone away by the time I was in the air. It was a new symptom, but I didn't dwell on it too much.

A month later, at the beginning of February 1997, I was back in Prague. I had asked to go for a coffee before heading off to the restaurant where Stefan had booked a table. My suspicions about him had grown, although it seemed unfair. He always rang when he promised to, he was amusing and charming during phone calls, and I enjoyed his company. My friends thought I was mad to be so cautious.

'It's important to be honest, Stefan,' I said looking at him, shocked again at how good-looking he was. 'If there's anything you want to tell me, go ahead. I shan't be angry.'

'No, there's nothing. Shall we go to the restaurant now?'

As we got into his car, he turned to me. 'You won't be angry?'

'No, I promise.'

'I have a girlfriend in the United States. I've been seeing her for four years.'

'Oh, I thought there was something.' I felt disappointed but I'd known my instincts about him were right. Thank God I hadn't taken it any further than friendship. But there was more to come.

'I have a girlfriend in Germany I've been seeing for two years. And a girlfriend in Prague whom I've known for six months.'

I burst out laughing. Thank goodness for gut feelings.

'Can I ask you one question? Was I going to be your London girl?'

'Yes, of course,' he said, without any embarrassment at all. His calm attitude touched a raw nerve.

'Take me back to my hotel, now!'

'What's your problem? I don't see what's wrong.'

We drove in silence and as we drew up at the hotel, he leaned over.

'Carole, you must understand. I have to make sure I find the right mother for my children.' My fit of temper had gone and I laughed out loud at that one.

'Well, it's definitely not me. Good luck in your search, Stefan.' I shook his hand and walked into the hotel lobby. My Prince Charming had turned out to be just a frog. The computer at work must have a heart for, by coincidence, I've never been back to Prague since.

Sara moved out of my flat at that time and for the first time since I had been single I was living alone. I didn't like it; what if I was taken ill during the night? But I didn't want a stranger moving in, so I stayed on my own.

Over the next few months I had different symptoms nearly every day. The burning sensation in my back came and went. Sometimes I had the feeling that sharp pins were being stuck into the sides of my face. Another time I jumped when I had the sensation of a spider crawling up my leg, but there was nothing there. One day, driving my car, I felt something hot dripping onto my foot. I pulled over and stopped to check but, again, there was nothing. Another day I had the sensation that the tops of my legs were hot, as though sun shining through the window was burning them. There was no sun on that March morning and when I touched my legs they felt cool.

Friends told me I should go to the doctor but my answer was always the same: 'What's the point? They can't do anything for me.' I didn't ignore the symptoms this time, though. I took a week off work and rested. I could tell by now when my body was warning me.

At Easter I went to Somerset to visit my dad. We spent the day on his boat around the coast at Torquay. Abi, my little sister, was ill with a tummy bug and Dad's wife Helena went down with it as the day went on. I started to feel unwell and as Dad drove us back to his house in Puriton I lay on the back seat of his car and slept.

I went to bed at 8.30 that evening. I tried to watch TV in my room but my eyes hurt so I went to sleep. Two hours later I was woken by shaking through my whole body. At first I thought I must be cold. I climbed out of bed – still shaking – and put on socks and a dressing gown and wrapped the quilt around me. As I lay down again and curled the quilt over me my head began to shake, too. I knew then that I wasn't shivering. My body had gone into spasm. This was definitely the MS.

I lay there for 20 minutes. The shaking stopped then started again. I was scared. I didn't want anybody to see me like this but I had to tell someone. What if it grew worse? I made my way downstairs. I was shaking so much I couldn't find my footing on the steps and my hand was unsteady on the bannister rail. I started to cry as the spasms went on and on. What if I was stuck like this? Oh please, don't let this be the start of a relapse.

Dad was watching TV and he leapt off the sofa as I appeared in the living-room doorway.

'What's the matter? What's happened?'

'I can't stop shaking, Dad. It's horrible.'

'Have you had a nightmare?' He put his arms around me and sat me down on the sofa. As he held me tight the spasm gradually calmed. Then it started up again. It seemed odd to be in this situation with my father. I can't ever remember cuddling him on the sofa; we'd never had that sort of relationship. It was always Mum who did that but I'm so glad he was there.

'This must really scare you, sweetheart,' he said. 'When things like this happen, I mean.'

'I'm scared now. Nothing quite like this has ever happened before.'

He put on the gas fire and I sat on the floor with my back to it. Then he made me a cup of tea.

'What do you think it is?' he asked.

'Maybe it's my reaction to the tummy bug. Don't worry. The chances are I'll wake up in the morning feeling fine.'

After about an hour the shaking eased slightly and I went to bed.

The next day I drove home. I was tearful and upset that my dad had seen me like that. I was annoyed with myself, too. I should have told my doctor about the strange symptoms I'd been having recently. That evening I could feel the spasms starting again, but they passed after only a flutter. It was enough to make me panic, though.

'You should have seen me before, Carole.' Dr Worthington looked worried, too. 'I want to examine you.'

'But what can you do? I'm just wasting your time. You could be seeing another patient!'

'I understand how you feel but you must let me log your symptoms. There may be a pattern to them.'

I was silenced. I'd never thought of that.

'I want you to see a neurologist. You've had a muscle spasm and I think this may be a relapse.' She phoned to make me an appointment.

I'd never classed symptoms as relapses. To me a relapse was something huge, like when I was taken ill in Rio. But I hadn't felt well since the previous October when I'd had my wisdom teeth removed. That was six months before and I'd had constant flu bugs, burning, tingling, and now this. I knew some people with MS had spasms every day, but I never had.

'The neurologist can see you in two months' time.' Dr Worthington smiled at me as she put down the phone.

'You see what I mean? I'll be fine by then! What's the point?'

16. The Employer's Story

Maggie Sheppard, 49, worked at British Airways for 27 years. She started as a stewardess and for her last eight years with the company was a Performance Manager. She is now a business training consultant and lives in Hampton, Middlesex. 'I wanted to manage Carole's situation so that everybody came out winning,' she says.

I managed 140 crew, of which Carole happened to be one. I already knew that she had multiple sclerosis because a colleague had told me and a condition such as that would be logged into our staff records. She came into my team because I was working on a Monday–Friday roster, which she went on, too. Carole needed the stability and support of her friends and having weekends off helped that. She also wanted consistency from her manager so she knew I would be at work on the same days as her.

She came to see me and I left it open to her to say what she could or couldn't cope with at work. At that stage she wasn't a special case. We always looked carefully at people who had regular sickness to see if there was a problem that we needed to deal with.

She asked me if I knew she had MS. Her manner at our first meeting, and most of the time since, was very ebullient and bouncy. She always gives off the message: 'I can cope'. When you look at Carole, it is easy to go into denial, to forget that she is ill. She adores her job and by reputation, and from personal experience through flying with her, she is excellent at her job. Passengers and her peers describe her as warm, friendly and outgoing. There is also a part of Carole that feels flying is normality for her. I think she sees leaving it, stepping outside of the job she knows and losing the security of colleagues, as a major difficulty.

My concern was that she wouldn't be able to maintain a high-energy, tiring job – either physically or mentally. It is an energetic job, lifting, getting up and down, and you're in the public eye all of the time. Normally our working days are 10–12 hours. I learnt to watch the effects of all this on her like a hawk.

When I met her I had a game plan in my head. First of all, I listened. I listened how this illness comes and goes. This was my only firsthand experience of managing someone with MS. I had managed other staff with chronic or terminal illnesses, but not MS. Years and years ago an old boyfriend's mother had MS so I knew how serious it could become. I became interested in what it does to people – what remission means, what effect stress has. I got my information from Carole herself and I read a report by the MS Society. I also talked to Dr Michael Bagshaw at BA for guidance, although he wasn't allowed to pass on any confidential information about Carole to me.

By our second meeting I felt she should be doing nine-hour days as a maximum. Whatever I did with Carole, I had to be careful that she went away and really thought about what she could do. I became the voice of caution and encouragement; she was sometimes over-ambitious about her energy levels. By our third meeting I said we needed to make some sort of career plan that gradually weaned her off flying. But I did mean gradually. We had other staff with chronic illnesses whose skills in other areas were built up so they could move on when the time became relevant. Carole sometimes seemed upset or cross about messages she didn't want to hear. I sensed a deep-seated frustration. Big changes like these are very sensitive issues. She felt she might be made to face up to something she didn't want to do.

She was relieved to have nine-hour duty days. But I had to tell her: 'We can't do this for ever and ever.' As management, we can't be seen to be more partial to one person than another. We're dealing with thousands of cabin crew on a daily basis so we can only adjust rosters for a certain amount of time, until a crisis is over, for example. My job was to make sure staff were able to maintain their job contracts. I wanted to manage Carole's situation so that everybody came out winning. All this has to be managed sensibly and with a heart, but it's also business. In my case, I had to keep staff in the air so the planes could fly.

Once I realized that even nine hours a day was hard for her to maintain then we had to have another discussion. I suggested I could help her to develop transferable skills, and we talked about public relations. I sensed resistance and uncertainty in her. It wasn't distrust, but more: 'Where is this conversation going to lead me?' Carole would say: 'Are you saying I'll have to leave?' My response was quite gentle. I'd say: 'Circumstances often drive decisions.' I wanted us to reach a consensus on what she could do.

Above all, I wanted Carole to work closely with me so she didn't feel that the unexpected was coming around the corner. There were about 17 supervisors in my team of cabin crew and I allocated Carole to Ian Few, a very paternal, kindly and popular man. But I was aware that whatever arrangements I made wouldn't last for long. Staff change and you can't maintain identical levels of support over a very long period. Carole was helped by her colleagues being extraordinarily supportive. Nobody ever came to me with any doubts about flying with her and there were never any 'tales told out of school' from other crew.

Even so, I had to take care not to make Carole a special case and not to over-allocate time. I had other people who were ill or in a crisis and in a small community like a company the even-handed use of time is paramount. You're always looking to the door of your office because you know someone else is waiting to be seen. When Carole is fixated on something she can demand a lot of time. Although I didn't ration it, I had to be careful not to be drawn along by her. Carole isn't ordinary; MS is not like other illnesses. One day she could be really well and the next chronically ill.

We counsel for ill-health retirement and it's a horrible tightrope to walk: we need to benefit the company and the person. Generally speaking, people realize themselves when they can't manage. But it's very different with MS, especially with someone as young as Carole. You're dealing with their life, emotions, aspirations. Every case is different which is what's so difficult about managing sick people. Some have husbands and families as a safety net. But how do you send someone who is single out of your office feeling disappointed or upset? A manager has to take that sort of thing into consideration.

Dealing with sickness within large companies is a lottery; some people are more rule-bound than others. I always had to explain any unusual work records, such as Carole's, to the Fleet Manager, who was my boss. If you're supporting someone through a bad patch at work you need to divulge something of their situation so that if you're off sick yourself, or away on holiday, they still have support. We had good communication between managers at BA so I could always keep the relevant people in the picture. But I'm very aware that being passed from manager to manager can be difficult. It can be embarrassing to explain your medical history or symptoms to someone else. It takes time to take people into your confidence and trust them. Perhaps a male steward would have found it difficult to come to me if he'd been diagnosed with prostate cancer.

As a manager you bring all your training and skills to bear when 'a Carole' walks through your door. I could always call on other managers' experience and expertize without giving away too many details of her situation, so I knew I had support in bearing the responsibility of steering Carole in the right direction. Equally, I had to remember how much BA had invested in her training and a company wants a return for that.

BA cabin services staff have to pass rigorous fitness tests because of the nature of their work. If she was on the ground, in some sort of administrative position, the decisions Carole has had to make might not be so dramatic. There is a cachet about putting on a uniform. A job like Carole's seems glamorous so any change from it is a big decision. I have a chronic back condition and had to take the decision to move away from full-time flying 18 years ago so I knew something of the thought processes Carole was going through. You have to be very fit to keep going as cabin crew. If you have anything wrong with you in cabin work, you go down like a ton of bricks. I'm saying that managing someone with MS could be very different in another walk of life.

I was very worried about Carole when she organized her first charity event. There was so much promotional work involved and she did far too much. But it led to her going on a course in public relations and marketing, so I knew that at least she was thinking about alternatives to flying.

It was my responsibility to prepare Carole for the time she'd stop flying but I wanted her to make the right decisions. Sometimes, I felt the process should be speeded up a little so that she didn't have to keep putting herself under any stress. I knew she was bright enough to know when she had to stop.

Managers are like everyone else, they are all different. Carole's career could have been very different if she had worked for another kind of manager. I'm not blowing my own trumpet. In fact, I was challenged gently by other colleagues about how much I was doing in Carole's case.

I was very aware of the care that must be taken so that an employee doesn't build up dependency on you. For example, some managers give their home phone numbers to lots of their staff, some to no one at all. You learn by experience how to deal with different people. I once found myself completely involved in a family's bereavement when a member of staff died. Having gone through that person's tears and anger I then had to go through the same with their spouse after the death. It taught me a valuable lesson. Carole had my home number but she never once abused it. Nor has she ever visited my house; we always drew a line between colleague and friend and we knew where we stood. All those decisions are very personal.

When you manage people you can be all things to them, but at the end of the day you are their manager. There is also a big personal risk. You can be rebuffed by staff because you're not giving them the answers they want, or you can be hauled over the coals by your own manager telling you to stop being so personally involved in a case. You have to assess who needs you the most and act accordingly.

You need to be very clear from the start with a person in Carole's circumstances. You must spell out what you can do within your remit, and what you can't. Maybe on our first few meetings I didn't do that with Carole. I don't know if anybody can be that incisive if they are dealing with someone's emotions as they approach a major turning point in their life. The easiest thing is to be 'Mr Nice Guy' but at some point you know you will reach a crucial situation and have to clamp down. In management, you have to look several steps ahead at all times.

I would say to other managers faced with 'a Carole' that the best thing is to sit and listen twice as hard as you'd listen to anyone else. You have to learn what they need or want from working life. They have the answers, you don't. Carole has the answer to how she moves to the future, I haven't. I can help, encourage, even give out advice – which I don't like doing – if I can see she is jumping in at the deep end. But you can never make anyone do anything.

I see great potential in Carole and a company could harness that potential. She has phenomenal energy, but only if she recognizes her limitations and sticks to them. If you can build up that special relationship with her, then she's a treasure in the workplace. But Carole, or whoever the ill person is, has to be part of any bargain; they have to be realistic about what they can do. Part of my deal with Carole was that she wouldn't come in to work if she felt ill. She broke that deal several times early on. But when she learnt that I would gladly help her, she rang the minute she felt ill and we all knew where we stood.

You have to be careful with Carole, perhaps with anyone with MS, because of the nature of the illness. She can almost hoodwink you by looking so well and bright. But she forces herself to be like that. It's a fragile bubble and I've seen it burst on several occasions, especially when Carole has been bereaved, tired or stressed in any way.

In recent years I've said to her several times: 'When will you realize that flying isn't the be-all and end-all of life? You can do other things.' I think Carole's future lies outside the airline. It could become a constant reminder of what she was, or what she could have been. I think she's moving on and she needs to be thinking of new beginnings. Anything is possible. I have grown very fond of Carole and wish that she could have a big, long remission from her MS. As for her future, I hope that she receives as much in life as she gives to others.

17. Letting Go of the Past

'How does it feel to be 30?' I was sitting in the garden of Henry J. Bean's, a restaurant in King's Road, Chelsea, on 6 April 1997. It was my birthday lunch. Ten of my girl friends were eating and chatting at a long wooden table and we were all drinking Pimm's. The sun was shining and I felt good. Sara had turned to me and asked the big question.

'Well, you already know, Sara!' I couldn't resist teasing her; she had hated turning 30.

'Seriously, Carole. How do you feel?' Sara's sister, Sofie, asked.

'Great! I know where I am and what I want from life.'

'What do you want?' This time it was Anna, a friend and fellow short-haul stewardess, who looked at me. I was sitting next to her on the arm of the wooden garden bench they were all sitting on. I started to sing.

'I tell you what I want, what I really, really want ...' They all groaned and we laughed.

'I want to keep healthy, I want to be happy and I want to settle down. I want to slow down, too.'

'Slow down? You!' Anna obviously didn't believe me.

'Seriously. I've decided not to organize a charity event this year. They take too much out of me on top of my job. I must focus on my health.'

'Do you want anything else?'

'I want to be a mum. It's just a case of finding the right dad! I can't do it on my own. Well, I suppose I could but I don't want to.'

It was good to come out of a spell of illness, to feel human again. I was finding work days more tiring but I was glad I'd shaken off the recent continual bouts of flu and colds. It was a chore to keep the appointment with the neurologist at St George's Hospital, Tooting. But I had taken notice of my doctor's warning that I needed to keep everyone in the picture.

A nurse did all the usual MS tests, checking reflexes, muscle strength, eyes, co-ordination. I knew them off by heart and knew that I was OK. She pulled out some needles to stick into my skin as a test of my sensitivity.

'Please don't stick that needle in me!' She laughed and put the needles away. I knew I didn't have numbness anywhere and it would hurt.

'You win. Can you feel this, though?' She brushed some cotton wool down my arm. Of course I could.

'How did I do?' I asked, not in the least bit worried.

'One thing concerns me slightly. By the way, there's a new neurologist here now, Dr Foster. He'll have a word with you.'

Dr Foster came into the consulting room, immaculate in a dark suit. We all sat down. He looked at my notes then at me.

'I'm amazed you can cope with the drive to Heathrow, let alone flying.'

He seemed to understand exactly how I felt. I was growing more and more concerned about the pressure my work was putting on me.

'Have you thought about taking ill-health retirement?'

'It has crossed my mind.'

'How would you feel about being a pensioner at your age? Would it upset you?'

'No. I'm just not ready yet. It does sound quite funny, though.'

'You really should have let me know about the symptoms you've been experiencing. It's important we have a record of them. You will keep in touch in the future, won't you?'

Dr Foster stood up, shook my hand and left. I turned to the nurse.

'What about the bit that concerned you?'

She ran after him and brought him back.

'I'm so sorry, Carole. There was something I should have talked to you about.'

He lapsed into doctor's jargon and I didn't have a clue what he was talking about.

'Can you stop, please. I don't understand what you're trying to say.'

'It appears that one of your eyes hasn't completely recovered from your first relapse.'

'I thought my eyes were fine. I haven't noticed any difference.'

He held out both arms with his wrists bent back, palms flat in front of my face.

'If you're normal your eyes can follow a finger being moved in front of them smoothly. One of your eyes is moving at a different pace to the other one. Like this.'

He moved both his arms to the left, one smoothly, one in small jerks so that I could see the difference. I was shocked. I had gone to the hospital feeling completely well.

As I drove home I understood why he had brought up the subject of a pension. It shook me that there was something wrong I hadn't known about. It made me self-conscious about my eyes. Blindness terrifies me. I have a horror of total blackness; it brings on a sense of claustrophobia. I know I would need someone with me all the time to keep that fear under control.

My job became an issue again. It was obvious that I couldn't keep flying forever. I was stuck in a vicious circle: bills, my health, needing rest, and losing pay when I took time off. The thought of not being a stewardess was hard for me but at least now I was listening to what everyone was saying. I phoned the BA doctor, Mike Bagshaw, to tell him about my eye problem.

'I trust you to let me know if there is any deterioration whatsoever in this condition,' he said. 'You could think about what your neurologist told you. Maybe you need to prepare yourself for ill-health retirement.'

'It has to be my own choice.'

'I know you'll make the right decision, Carole.'

It was our same old bargain but it seemed more urgent now.

Everyone was pressing me to think about the future. The time for change seemed to be drawing closer.

In May Anna moved into my flat. I had met her at my friend Maxine's house when we had sat nattering until dawn and we'd been friends ever since. She had split up with her boyfriend and wanted somewhere to stay until she was back on her feet. I was pleased to have someone around.

But the weekend she moved in, an old schoolfriend from Banff died. I couldn't believe it as I flew up to Scotland. Gail was attractive, kind, funny. She was a perfectionist, too. I smiled as I remembered her in school uniform, obsessed with making sure both her socks were pulled up to exactly the same height. A few days earlier, she had hanged herself.

Her family was devastated. They had asked six of her old friends to visit them the night before the funeral, which was to be for family only. It was heartbreaking. Afterwards we all gathered at Lorraine's house. She was one of the group and I was staying with her. I was the only one of us who had moved away. Most of them were married with children but that evening all we wanted was to sit and talk over old times.

I flew home a few days later feeling desperately sad. Gail had been surrounded by friends but had taken her own life. If only I had phoned her. If only she had phoned me to talk through whatever was troubling her. The sheer waste of life made me weep.

Anna was at my flat to meet me, her eyes anxious when she saw how upset I was. There was a message on the answer phone from my friend Sofie, too.

'I don't know how you're feeling, Carole, but it's Ronnie Wood's birthday party tonight. Would you like to go? Give me a call.'

I could think of nothing worse.

'It might do you good to think about something else,' Anna said. 'It's too good an opportunity to miss.'

'I'm really not in a party mood, Anna.'

'Sofie would love you to go with her.'

A few hours later I was driving along a street in Kingston, London.

Sofie was in the passenger seat and we were trying to find the party. Ahead we spotted crowds of people behind metal barriers and a separate crowd of press photographers.

'That must be it,' Sofie said. I knew Ronnie Wood was one of the Rolling Stones, but I'd been a punk as a teenager and the Stones had never meant much to me. The crowd surprised me. Sofie's brother, Steve, was a friend of Ronnie Wood's son, which is why we were on the guest list.

As I drew nearer a security man came round to my side of the car. I wound down the car window as he searched for our names on his list.

'I'll park your car, madam. Just go straight through the gate over there.' He pointed into the dark as I gave him my car keys and stepped out of the car. Dozens of cameras clicked and flashed and all I could see was dots in front of my eyes. I was still blinded when I heard Sofie's brother laughing at the other side of the gate. I realized why celebrities wear sunglasses at night. It isn't for their image, it's for protection!

'What a waste of their film!' I shouted across to Steve, wondering who the press thought would turn up at such a glamorous event in an old Volkswagen Golf like mine.

Steve gave us both a hug as we walked into the driveway. We entered the Wild West. Ronnie Wood had chosen a Cowboys and Indians theme for his fiftieth birthday party. There was straw on the ground and hay bales scattered around as seats. Most of the guests were in costume, some firing toy guns into the air. A wild boar roasted on a spit and guests whooped with laughter as they tried to stay on a bucking bronco machine. An enormous green-and-white-striped marquee opened down to the back garden. It was so huge that it hid the house. All I could see was one turret silhouetted against the dark sky.

There were security men everywhere, their ear-phones wired to walkie-talkies. They mingled with the hundreds of people standing in groups, chatting and sipping drinks. We were each given a glass of champagne and wandered into the part of the marquee set up as a cash-free casino. Formula One world champion Damon Hill and his wife Georgie were trying their luck at roulette. A croupier in a striped waistcoat, a green visor shading her eyes, was spinning the wheel. I looked at Sofie.

'Let's go and mingle,' I said as I began to take in some of the famous faces around us. 'And Sofie, I'm not going to talk about Gail tonight.'

Sofie put her arm round my shoulder. 'You can if you want to. I'll listen.'

Our last-minute decision meant we weren't in costume, but the guests who were looked stunning. The first face we recognized was Texan model Jerry Hall, fabulous in her cream leather cowgirl outfit and enormous Stetson hat. Her husband Mick Jagger – the only other Rolling Stone I would recognize – was with her.

'Look who's over there.' Sofie nodded towards a corner of the marquee and there was Mick Hucknall of Simply Red.

'Let's sit down,' I said. We found some spaces at one of the wooden tables near the casino. We realized that we were sharing it with Noel Gallagher, his fiancée Meg Mathews, supermodel Kate Moss and Jools Holland. They smiled and shuffled along the wooden benches to make room. Then Steve walked over with a young man with blond hair tied into a ponytail and bright blue eyes.

'I'd like you to meet Jamie,' Steve said introducing us to Ronnie Wood's son. We all stood chatting and laughing and Jamie's girl-friend, Charlotte, joined us.

'Here come Mum and Dad,' Jamie said a little later. 'Move up and we can all sit together.'

'Are you having a good time?' Ronnie asked us as his wife, Jo, sat down next to me. I didn't feel in the least starstruck with them; they just seemed a really nice family.

'Yes, it's great. Happy birthday!'

'Just you wait till the fireworks!'

Ruby Wax, in scarlet, walked over for a chat with Ronnie and actor John Hurt joined in. Then there was a gasp from people at the other side of the marquee. We all craned our necks and the most incredible cake I have ever seen was wheeled onto the dance floor. Six feet wide, it was a model of the family home on one side, with sugar models of each member sitting on the windowsills. The other side was decorated as a Wild West saloon, bank and jailhouse. It was a work of art.

After it was cut and everybody sang 'Happy Birthday', Ronnie Wood shouted: 'Everybody follow me down to the tennis courts!' As we walked, glasses in our hands, there was an explosion of noise and colour as a firework display began.

Later, back in the marquee, Ronnie leapt onto the stage and started to sing Country and Western songs. He was joined by Marianne Faithfull and Tim Rice, with Jools Holland playing an electric organ. It was magical.

I looked around the marquee and let my mind wander.

'Sofie.' I leaned over and whispered to her. 'Think of the concert I could put together just with the people in this room.'

'God, that would be amazing, Carole.'

'This is a private party. I can't ask them now. If we were somewhere else I would.'

I leant back in my chair. In my head I had a picture of Wembley Stadium, sold out for one of the biggest rock concerts ever and hundreds of thousands of pounds being raised for MS research. It would be a dream come true.

We danced till the early hours. Jamie introduced me to one of his friends, Liam, who had green eyes and the sweetest smile. We sat talking for hours. I told him all about Gail, even though I'd told Sofie that I didn't want to talk about her at all. We discussed my MS and he listened, quietly. I told him my life story, I suppose. He told me his, too. Then I noticed it was 6 a.m.

'I have to go home or I'll drop. I had no idea of the time.'

'Would you give me a lift? You go past where I live,' Liam asked.

I made several friends that evening, and it was the first of many visits to the Woods' home. As Sofie, Liam and I made our way down the drive, Jo and Ronnie Wood came walking towards us.

'Thanks for a great party,' I said, and kissed them both on the cheek.

'It's all right for some!' Ronnie shouted. Liam laughed as he realized he was leaving the party with a girl on each arm.

Three days later, on 4 June 1997, I was driving past Wimbledon football stadium on my way to visit a friend with my car radio on.

'Rock star Ronnie Lane, one of the founder members of The Small Faces, died today after a 20-year battle against multiple sclerosis. He was 51.'

I had never heard of him, but anything mentioning MS made me listen hard. Then Ronnie Wood and Rod Stewart were each mentioned. I hadn't known they were all in The Faces together. I phoned Sofie on my mobile.

'Don't you think it's strange? I had no idea Ronnie Wood had any experience of knowing someone with MS. Did you?'

'No. It seems a weird coincidence, though, just after you met him.'

The MS Society told me they were getting phone calls and letters about the TV documentary I'd done. It confirmed an idea I'd had months ago. Why not turn my bit of the programme into a short video for people newly-diagnosed with MS? All I needed was sponsorship. I set up a meeting between Channel Four, which had screened the programme, British Airways and the MS Society.

While I was organizing all of that, my friend Denise left me a note at work. 'Dear Carole, I've forgotten what your feet look like! We've got to get together soon. I miss you. Love, Denise.' She was right; we'd been trying to organize lunch for ages. I hadn't had reflexology for months, either. My meeting about the video was due later that week, on the Thursday, so I put her note in my pocket and decided to phone her afterwards.

'I can remember how I felt when I was diagnosed with MS.' I looked around the table in the conference room at Heathrow. Everyone nodded sympathetically. 'If I'd had someone else to relate to, or heard someone else's story, that would have helped a lot. I'd like to have heard about someone eight years down the line who is still getting on with her life. If I had known that she had learnt to live with it, then I'd have had more hope, too. Perhaps this video could take away that sense of loneliness from just one person. I can't do anything else. It's up to you to make that happen.'

I sat down. After very little discussion BA offered to sponsor the venture and Channel Four agreed to make 5000 copies of the video. That meant it would go to people with MS free of charge, which was exactly what I'd wanted. The programme would be used to help others instead of gathering dust in a TV library somewhere. I left the room and felt so pleased that I burst into tears.

I meant to phone Denise with the good news but I forgot. The next Monday I had a Manchester night-stop and in the crew was Sue Johnston, her long, blonde hair stylishly plaited in a French twist. She was a good friend of Denise's, too. When we touched down in Manchester, Sue and I went out for a meal. The flight hadn't been long enough for all the chatting we needed to do to catch up with each other.

'We must all get together soon,' I said, after I'd told her about Denise's note to me. 'Take my number, Sue, just in case you've lost it.'

'Don't forget to sort it out. We've gone too long without seeing each other.'

We had the red-eye flight back to Heathrow the next morning and I was home by 9.30 a.m. I put on a pot of coffee, retrieved the remote control from the back of the sofa and flicked on the TV. Kilroy was on. Then the phone rang. It was Sue Johnston.

'Carole, have you read the *Daily Mail*?'

'No. Why?'

'I'm sorry. I've got the most devastating news for you.'

She sounded calm. All I could think as Sue began to read from the paper was: What could possibly be in it which would have anything to do with me? Then I froze as she read out: ' Denise Rothwell, 32, was killed on Sunday night when her car crashed into a Scottish river ...'

'It's not true, it can't be.'

'It's here in the paper, Carole. I can't believe it either.'

'I'll phone BA. Someone there will know.' I dialled the office but Maggie, my own manager, wasn't there. Another one came on the line.

'That's right, Carole. Denise was killed on Sunday night.' As she spoke I broke down. Sobbing and not really knowing what I was doing, I rang Sue back immediately. I came off the phone and forced myself to calm down before ringing my flatmate, Anna, on her mobile. She was on the train, coming home from Heathrow.

'Anna, could you pick up a copy of the Daily Mail somewhere?'

'Sure. Are you OK, Carole?'

'Yes, I'm fine.'

By the time she arrived I was sobbing. As she walked through the door and saw me, she dropped her overnight case and handbag.

'Oh God, what's wrong?'

I couldn't speak. She sat next to me on the sofa. I picked up the paper from the floor where she'd dropped it, sat back down and found the page about Denise. I let out another sob. As Anna realized what had happened she put her arms around me and I wept.

I lay on the sofa, staring at the ceiling. Why should Denise die? She had everything to live for. I was too shocked to think about the details of the accident. There was even a photograph of the mangled car after it had been dredged from the river.

Then the phone began to ring. First my manager, Maggie. Then the MS Society, Channel Four, everyone who had been involved with Denise and me on the video. It went on and on. Within three hours, the press started to call as well. My name was on file with Denise from the publicity we'd done for the TV programme. They had looked her up when the news of the crash had come through and discovered they had photographs of the two of us together. They wanted to use them. What could I say? I wanted her to be remembered for the wonderful person she was. Each time I spoke about her, I broke down again.

I decided to go into work the next day. It was no good sitting on the sofa, sobbing. Work usually takes my mind off things. I was rostered for a return trip to Manchester and I couldn't have asked for a better crew. They all knew Denise and I had been friends, and all the newspapers with our picture in were removed from the plane. The ground staff weren't so understanding on the return flight and all the papers were brought onto the aircraft.

I was standing between two trolleys in the aisle when I glanced up and saw a huge picture of Denise smiling at me from the page of a newspaper. I turned around and another passenger was holding up a paper which had the picture of the two of us. I panicked. I had to get out of there. A stewardess moved the trolley aside and I walked into the galley before breaking down in tears. I cried all the way home. It was no good. I wasn't ready for work yet.

I was back on a plane for a funeral in Scotland, less than two months after Gail's. This time it was Glasgow. My sister Hazel took me to the airport in the morning where I met three stewards, Mark, Ollie and Nelson. The four of us were her closest friends at BA but we had never met each other.

Mark had come straight off a flight from Tel Aviv and was still in his uniform. We sat together, trying desperately to keep a conversation going without breaking down, but when we landed in Glasgow we all fell quiet. None of us wanted to be there and we knew the next few days would be hard.

We booked into the Glasgow Marriott hotel. Mark and I sat talking, chain-smoking our way through the hours until the first funeral service, to be held that evening.

'If Denise could see us now, smoking like this, she'd kill us!' Mark said, his blue eyes red-rimmed with sadness and tiredness.

'How did you meet Denise, Mark?'

'On an Amsterdam night-stop, four years ago. Don't laugh. I felt she had an aura about her. She was so selfless. She always made me feel good about myself. Do you know what I mean?'

'It really upsets me that it's her death that has brought all of us together.' I started to cry. Gail and Denise; their faces flashed through my mind. I would never see them again. It just didn't seem real.

It was a small, Catholic service at St Philomena's, Glasgow, and a second service was held the next morning. Then we made our way to the crematorium for her cremation. I was exhausted and only just keeping myself together. When members of her family came over and referred to me by name it took me some time to realize that they had recognized me from the TV documentary. I wasn't functioning properly at all.

We all flew home together, dressed in black and barely able to speak. Hazel picked me up and once I was in the car, I lost control. She gently held my hand, steering with the other, as I sobbed and tried to talk about Denise.

This time I couldn't cope. I went home and went to pieces. I didn't even have the energy to get dressed, let alone go to work. I was trying to find a reason for these two young deaths. What was the point of Gail or Denise dying? It made me angry, upset, then angry again. Every now and then I would take out the note Denise had written me a few days before her death, and cry. I sat clutching the video of the documentary. Part of me wanted to watch it so that I could see Denise's face and hear her voice. I couldn't do it, though. I phoned Mum.

'This is so hard,' I said.

'I know, sweetheart. I wish I could say something to help.'

'But why should they die? What's the point, mum?' I cried and cried.

'Is Anna there with you, darling?'

'No. I'm on my own. She's at work.'

'I wish I could be with you.'

I thought back to my last charity event. I'd spoken to Denise for five minutes all evening. If I could have that time again, she'd have been at my side all the time. I was just too busy that night. I thought of all the meetings we'd postponed. Our lives were so hectic that for months all we'd do was speak on the phone. I began ringing my friends. If Denise and Gail could die just like that, so could anyone else. I needed them all to know how much I loved them.

The July and August issues of *Zest* health magazine landed on my doormat during this period at home. They carried a two-part, very upbeat interview with me, written months earlier. In the smiling photograph I looked confident and relaxed. It was like staring at a stranger.

I rang the BA doctor, Mike Bagshaw. I felt he ought to know what was happening as it was part of our deal to keep me flying.

'The truth is, Dr Bagshaw, I'm not coping very well.' I was sitting in my dressing gown looking dreadful, but my voice was calm.

'I don't think anybody would be able to cope with all this. I want you to do something for me.'

'Of course. What?'

'I want you to talk to our counselling service.'

'No. I'd be too worried that it would get around the company.'

'That won't happen, I can promise you.'

I trusted Dr Bagshaw so I rang the counselling office. A receptionist answered.

'Would you like to see someone regarding illness, bereavement, work or relationships?'

'All of them, please,' I replied. I didn't mean it as a joke; I felt that everything around me was falling apart.

I was assigned to Arthur, a kind, softly-spoken Glaswegian. I assumed I would talk about Gail or Denise but discovered it was too early, the grief was still too new. Instead, he took me back to my diagnosis with MS, my grandfather's death, Craig leaving me, all the milestones of the past eight years.

'You know, Carole, death, broken relationships and illness are all losses. You've lost a lot for someone of your age.' I had never looked at it like that before. By my fourth session with Arthur I'd had another idea.

'I'd like to counsel people with MS so that they'd have someone who understood to listen to their problems.'

'Well, you stumbled through the period after your own diagnosis and seem to have found a way of accepting it.'

'I would need training. I don't know how to guide people in the right direction.'

He gave me the addresses of several training courses.

Three weeks after Denise's funeral I returned to work. The atmosphere wasn't good. Cabin crew had been on strike while I'd been off sick and everyone was on edge. On my first flight, which was to Hamburg, I took it all out on a passenger, for the first time since I'd been flying.

I was walking through the cabin handing out newspapers when a youngish businessman asked me for the *Financial Times*. I didn't have any left. Instead of asking for another paper, he lost his temper.

'What do you mean, there are no *FT*s? It's a disgrace.'

'Sir, is it that important that you get the *FT*?'

'Yes, it is.'

'Then may I suggest that the next time you board an aircraft you buy one in the terminal so you can have your own?'

I walked away. I knew I was wrong but after my recent experiences he seemed unbelievably petty. Later in the flight I found a used copy of the *FT* and gave it to him. I had to appreciate that I had no idea what his background was. Perhaps going without his newspaper had been the final straw for him, too. He could have reported me but he didn't and I was glad. I've got a clean slate at BA, no customer has ever complained about me, and I would like to keep it that way.

Anna moved out at this time into a house nearby. I was on my own again but I had a good circle of close friends who were all only a phone call away. My previous fears about being alone at night were fading away.

In the meantime I was making inquiries about training as a counsellor as my sessions with Arthur came to an end. If I built up a good case before I saw my manager I thought she would be more likely to say yes. I found that most course tutors weren't happy about taking on someone who'd suffered recent bereavements, but a few said they would. I went to Barbados at the end of August, to lie in the sun and think about my future.

Two days after I arrived at the Almond Beach village resort, Princess Diana was killed. I was on holiday in one of the most beautiful spots in the world and surrounded by people discussing the death of a young woman in a car crash. Denise flooded my mind. Even so, after a few days I found myself feeling more and more relaxed. I would lie by the pool, eat, try out lots of different cocktails, and go kayaking every afternoon. It was a resort for couples, though. It made me think of all the places I still want to visit: Mauritius, Bermuda, Hawaii, the Seychelles. Not Rio, though. I don't particularly want to go back there. But they're all places I'd want to go to with a man – just like Barbados! My job gives me the gift of cheap travel and I hadn't been making the most of it since I'd been single. I realized that I wanted someone to share it with.

As we took off on the flight home, which was the day of the Princess's funeral, the captain asked for a minute's silence. I looked out of the window; I had never heard complete silence on an aircraft before and as we dipped over the island then left it behind I made a decision: I would become a counsellor.

'I know exactly what I'm going to do with my life.' My manager, Maggie, looked at me from the other side of her desk. She listened as I outlined my plan for training as a counsellor in preparation for leaving BA. She didn't say a word.

'You don't think I should be doing this, do you?'

'No, I don't.'

We had a heated discussion. It wasn't an argument; Maggie and I never argued. But we frequently disagreed, particularly about my future.

'Why won't you support me, Maggie?'

'You'll be drained in work like that. You won't be able to detach yourself, however good your training is. I don't doubt that you could do it, you've got empathy and ability. But please, do yourself a favour.'

I was shocked but went away and thought hard. I saw her a week later.

'You're right, Maggie. I couldn't detach myself. I'd worry about my clients for weeks after their visits. It wouldn't be good for my health.'

I wanted to share my experiences, particularly in my fight to accept MS. I had so much to offer, but how could I do it? At about that time I saw Hugh Whitworth, who had directed the TV documentary I had been in, for lunch.

'You know, Carole, there's a book in you. You should tell your story,' he said after I'd described my efforts to find a life for myself beyond flying.

'Yeah, I'm sure. And how could I write a book?'

'Find a ghostwriter.'

I went back to Maggie.

'I don't want to work in public relations, I can't become a counsellor. I want to write a book. It might help someone else in my situation.'

'I think that's an excellent idea. But don't take on more than you can cope with, and *remain detached*.'

'I've thought of that. I shall ask someone else to write it for me.'

I went back to Australia for Christmas and New Year and this time my visit was very different. I felt healthier and stronger than I'd been for a long while and my mind was at rest. I was still flying but I knew that would have to stop some time and I was beginning to accept that. I felt that at last I was moving in the right direction.

Mum and Ivan wanted to make it a New Year's Eve party to remember. We spent hours peeling a sinkfull of fresh prawns so that Ivan could make his famous chilli prawns on the barbecue. We put balloons everywhere with tables and chairs dotted around the pool and the garden. The house started to fill up with family, friends, and neighbours. There was even an old schoolfriend of mine from Banff; by one of those incredible coincidences, she was marrying an Australian and settling nearby. Mum introduced me to her new neighbour, whose house was still being built. It turned out that she was a reflexologist.

'You seem to know a lot about reflexology, Carole,' she said as we went into the subject deeper and deeper.

'I had a friend who did it. She was killed in a car crash this summer. I haven't had it since.'

'Perhaps the next time you're in Australia, if you feel ready, I could do it for you?'

'Maybe.' Yes, that would be a good idea. It was time to look forward.

I stood staring into the swimming pool, hardly noticing the guests who were splashing around to cool down on this hot, hot night. I couldn't wait for 1998. I wanted 1997 to be over so that I could really move on. I hadn't felt like that at the end of a year for a long time.

I had phoned my dad and my sister, who were together in Somerset, earlier. One of the things I hate about New Year is that there's always somebody missing, especially when parents are divorced. But this was a good party and I wasn't going to waste it by thinking like that. I breathed in and smiled, at nobody in particular.

'You look happy, sweetheart.' My mum walked towards me, a glass of champagne in her hand. We linked arms, both of us wanting to make the most of being together on this lovely evening. Just then, Ivan put on the radio at full volume and cheering flooded the garden as the countdown to midnight began. Six, five, four, three, two ... Happy New Year! Everyone was shouting and laughing and hugging one another. Mum turned to me, smiling. 'I've got a feeling 1998 will be a good year for you, darling.'

'I hope so, Mum.'

'Have you made a New Year's resolution?'

'Yes, I have. I want to let go of the past and make the most of every single moment of my future.'

18. What will be, will be

As my mother always says: 'Que sera, sera, What will be, will be ...'

Unfortunately my New Year's resolution had to be postponed as I relived the hardest four years of my life by working on this book. It was as though I went into character; I had moments of anger, fear and tears. When I got to Australia in the book to be with my mother I actually started to feel better in real life.

There were moments when I needed time alone and moments when I desperately needed my friends around me. I needed their support so much while I was working on this book, and believe me I got it. There were times when I wondered whether it was worth putting myself through this. That only happened twice and they didn't last long. On both occasions I was contacted by strangers.

One wrote me a letter. She lived in Vienna and had seen my video. It was as if she wanted me to be her voice. Meanwhile, she was on her own private awareness campaign in Vienna. The next time was the day we spent on interviews about my grandfather. I still miss him desperately. There were a few tears that day and I was emotionally exhausted. So was my ghost-writer Sue!

I sat down at the end of the day and the phone rang. It was a lady from Leicester whom I'd spoken to once before when she had contacted me after seeing the Channel Four TV documentary. She came on the phone and began sobbing almost immediately about the way her family refuses to believe she has MS. She could hardly see as she was having problems with her eyesight and yet still her family put so many demands on her. She felt that I was the only person in the world that she could talk to and I was the only person who could understand what she was going through, even though we were strangers.

She spent half-an-hour sobbing about her MS and her family's denial. She just kept saying: 'Nobody understands what it's like.' But I did, and she knew that. She then apologised for not asking how I was. I told her not to be sorry and that she was right, most people don't understand. I explained to her that before she called I was having doubts about the book as it all seemed too painful. Her call reminded me why I wanted to write this book, to help other people understand. If we achieve some level of understanding, it will be worthwhile. I thought at first that her timing couldn't have been worse. In fact, it couldn't have been better and I never had doubts again.

When someone is diagnosed with an illness, the focus is always on them. What we forget is how it affects the people around them, their family, their friends. But sometimes it is difficult for them to understand when it's an illness they can't see.

For a person with MS the illness is like a shadow that you live with every single day of your life. It's always there but you can't always see it. It appears when you least expect it but you never know what form it's going to take or how long it's going to last. Also, other people don't always notice that it's there. It's too easy to lie about symptoms when they're not visible. You can tell people you're fine. Meanwhile your legs could be tingling, you could have numbness appearing and you could be terrified of the possibility of a relapse.

On the other hand, not everyone believes you when you do tell them. I've come across that several times in the eight years since my diagnosis. Not everyone even believes that you have MS, although that is quite rare. It is so frustrating if people think you are pretending to be tired or faking a symptom.

During the writing of this book I was in a car accident and had to wear a surgical collar. People showed enormous concern about my well-being at that time. In fact, that was the least of my problems. I was more worried about the things you couldn't see. The burning sensations, which grew worse and worse, the numbness, the heaviness in my legs, which then led to a relapse.

I know that symptoms can be used by some people to manipulate those closest to them. I could never pretend to have symptoms. For me it would be tempting fate. Also it would worry my family and friends unnecessarily and I would never play with their emotions like that. I admit that in the past I have lied and pretended about not having any symptoms. I felt that what people didn't know wouldn't hurt them. Now I realize that it hurts them more to think I am not being honest. I now tell those close to me about my symptoms, not every single little one, but the ones that worry me. If I have numbness in my leg one day I will keep quiet. But if it's still there when I wake up the next morning, or it has spread in any way, then I will tell someone.

I think you really have to want to be healthy and well to live with MS. You really have to want to get better. Sometimes things are too much of an effort, but it's important to me to make that effort. I hate being ill. I hate being stuck at home. And I hate going to the doctor. For me, it's a bit like a card game. Each individual player must accept the cards that life deals, but once they're in your hand it's up to you how you play them. My choice is to try and win the game.

The unpredictability of my illness is by far the hardest psychological burden. I know that if I'm well today, I may be ill tomorrow. And if I'm ill, will it turn into a relapse, or will I go from relapsing/remitting MS into the progressive form of the illness?

There were six points about the period before I was diagnosed with MS which troubled me the most:

1. Not knowing what was wrong for three months
2. Doctors, neurologists, specialists knowing and not telling me
3. The feeling that perhaps it was just in my head
4. I should have been told sooner
5. I deserved the whole truth from the medical profession
6. I could have dealt with anything if I'd known what I was dealing with.

The same six points about the manner in which Craig left me caused me the most pain as well:

1. Not knowing what was going on for two months
2. Everyone knew except me
3. I began to think my suspicions were just in my head
4. I deserved to be told sooner
5. I deserved the whole truth
6. I could have dealt with it had I known what I was dealing with.

I wanted answers on both occasions but I got traumatic answers. I now realize why I hate not knowing. Honesty is the best policy. These events have taught me to demand honesty and made me realize how important it is for me to be honest. Not just with other people, but also to myself. Sometimes the truth hurts and sometimes it's difficult for people to give me the honesty I would like from them. If someone wants an honest answer to a question from me, they'll get it. I will be the one to decide if I can or can't deal with the truth.

When I met Craig communication was not at the top of my wish-list in a man. Having MS has made things very different for me. I need to have communication and it has to work both ways. Craig and I were very young and we were dealt some bad deals. I wasn't easy to live with at that time, either. But as a friend he is now very supportive and I know we will always remain friends. The man for me must have the strength to deal with MS, no matter what, and be positive about life. I'd rather be single and happy than unhappy in a relationship. I do have moments of loneliness, mostly at night-time. I miss having someone to cuddle.

While I was working on this book during 1998, I did meet someone special who taught me that I am capable of loving again. There was a time when I didn't think I would ever let those barriers down. But I panicked and didn't know what to do. Love is an emotion you cannot control and that scared me. I realize now that I wasn't ready; in fact, neither of us was ready. But instead I've gained a very special friend.

You can't move forward in life unless you let go of the past.

Sometimes it is hard to let go but you have to, otherwise it holds you back. This book has proved to be a cathartic experience for me. It has helped me to leave the bad memories behind and take only the good memories with me into the future. Sometimes love hurts but with the wisdom of hindsight the one thing I know now is that it will never hurt so much as the first time and I will get over it. I came through it once and I will come through it again.

The book has given me understanding and realization of events in my life. It has made me realize that everything in life is temporary. Nothing lasts forever. The death of friends and members of my family has made me realize just how brief life is. You don't get a second chance. It has given me a different perception of life. You have to enjoy it while you can and I have every intention of living my life to the full. I believe that life is a learning process and when we die we use our knowledge and experience to guide others. I believe we become angels. I'm sorry if that makes me sound wacky, but it's my way of accepting death. For me, it takes some of the pain away. I can think of no other explanation for how unpredictable and final it is. Maybe that's why I hate goodbyes so much. 'See you later' doesn't seem so final.

Throughout these tragic events I have had the support of my friends and I don't know what I would do without them. I am very aware that not everyone is lucky enough to be surrounded by friends. When you're diagnosed with an illness like MS and you don't have your family living nearby, it means relying heavily on friends. I also had to get my priorities sorted out. Health has to come top and sometimes that means letting people down or missing out on something I want to do. I haven't given up anything completely but just do everything in moderation. Someday perhaps I will stop smoking, but that's my only vice. Listening to your body is the best guide to well-being and good health. It never lies to you.

MS does not mean that my life has come to an end. In fact, for me, it was a new beginning. It means that I have needed to adapt to a new lifestyle that suits my own limits and capabilities. When I was in Australia I had time to exercise, swim, and concentrate on my diet to be healthy. As you can see, I've been very busy in the last few years and it has been difficult to find the time.

However, you have to make time. I find meditation very important for my own well-being and I can always find the time for that. There are so many things that I intend to do. Alternative therapies are obviously very important to me. I also plan to embark on a new exercise programme, a mixture of T'ai Chi and yoga, which I've wanted to do for a long time. For me, it's also very important to have a daily intake of all the vitamins I need for day-to-day living.

I've had a cleaner for the last three years. Her name is Julie and I don't know what I'd do without her. She only comes once a fortnight but cleaning my flat really was too much for me on top of my job. I found that after scrubbing the bathroom my whole body would be shaking. The money I spend on her is money well spent. Again, it's about getting your priorities right. If it came to paying her or going out for an evening, then I'd plump for the cleaner every time. I don't see her as a luxury; I see her as a necessity in my life. However, it is not all about helping me. Friendship works both ways. As much as I need friends in my life, it is also important that they always know I am there for them. MS does not affect my hearing so I am always there to listen. I would hate for them to feel they couldn't come to me for support because I have MS. That would hurt me more but I understand why they may feel they can't put me under any extra pressure or stress. I want them to be able to come to me.

Fortunately I am surrounded by friends who are very positive about life. But it's hard to be positive when you're having a relapse. I don't think people have any idea how scared you feel; not knowing if it's going to debilitate you totally this time around, which part of your body will be affected, or how long the relapse will last. Severity is different for everyone. MS is individual, no two cases are exactly the same so each person diagnosed with MS has to work out for themselves what is best for them. If only we could put positive thinking in a bottle.

It took me a long time to learn to be positive. The first four years after I was diagnosed I was very angry that I had MS. I was angry because I was so young and a big chunk of my youth had been taken away from me. I was 23 when I was first taken ill in Rio. I was doing a job I loved and I was in party mode – then I was stopped in my tracks. It seemed so unfair.

Now I realize that being angry was a waste of energy. I kept thinking: 'Why me? Why MS?' It took those four years for me to turn that around and think 'Why not me?' Although I don't feel angry any more I still find it frightening, but most of all I find it frustrating. My mind will want to do one thing and my body will want to do another. It's a constant battle between the two. My body can't always keep up and sometimes I have no choice but to stop everything and rest. That is when the frustration sets in. I feel I have so much to do in life but not enough time to do it. And then some of that time is taken away from me by my illness. I think that's what makes me impatient about life.

Unfortunately I have also encountered jealousy. I find that very hard to comprehend as I feel some people miss the point. I would give up everything to have my health back. I don't understand how anybody could be jealous of someone having MS – I wouldn't wish it on my worst enemy. Luckily, it is not an emotion I have experienced very often. I find it very sad, as jealousy is so destructive. I can only admire people who do well in life. I like to see people happy.

I can think of two examples. At work, I'm on a restricted roster so my workload is obviously much easier than most of my colleagues. But I would love to be able to work a full roster. The other issue is my car, which I was given by Motability, which is a charity, after an assessment by my doctor. I have that car because it makes my life easier. Some days I have difficulty getting around. On bad days, if my co-ordination is poor or my arms and legs feel weak, I can't even turn the steering wheel or operate the clutch. I can insure it for other people to drive so that on those days, or if I'm in a relapse, I still have the freedom to move around. I have that car because I have multiple sclerosis. Which would you chose?

Everyone has the right to their own opinion. We forget that, as with any illness, MS also affects the people around them. I wanted my ex-boyfriend, mum, dad and manager to be completely honest about how my MS has affected them. As I have said, when someone is diagnosed the focus is on the person with the illness. I know it was difficult for them to relive certain times and to talk so openly, sometimes for the first time, about things they may prefer to forget or not even think about. I think they were all very honest and very brave and it has been a good process to bring everything out into the open. I have found it extremely difficult and sometimes painful to hear what they have to say but it has also given me understanding.

I want everyone to appreciate how complex close relationships are and how differently people react to something like an illness. It has been a strange process but it has been worth it. It has given all of us an understanding. Communication is vital; without it you don't have any real understanding. It's up to the person with MS to tell their family and friends how their MS makes them feel.

This is also important in the workplace. Flying was a dream come true for me. I've been all over the world in the past 10 years and met some wonderful people. My God, crew know how to party! And I will leave with happy memories. It is hard work, glamour and grind in equal measures. But it is becoming too much for me now. The thought of giving up flying has always worried me. I would miss the security of BA and the support of my colleagues. It used to make me angry and frustrated when people broached the subject. I felt it would be giving in to the MS and letting it take control of my life. It wasn't just my manager, Maggie, that I felt angry with when she mentioned not flying, but also my friends. I felt as though they all thought I couldn't cope. Sometimes they were right, but I wanted to cope desperately.

For me, flying was my life, my only normality. It was hard to accept that I was finding it difficult to get to work every day. The drive to Heathrow was bad enough in itself some days, let alone actually doing my job. The first person to bring it up with me was my friend Maxine's husband, Paul. He timed it just right and I finally accepted I was finding work a struggle, that I always felt so tired. It was getting very difficult to get up at 4 a.m., then drive to Heathrow and serve the public with a smile on my face. My body was telling me something and maybe it was time to listen.

I felt sad once I'd admitted how I felt but I was surprised to find that it wasn't a question of losing control, but rather of acceptance. It meant that I could plan ahead. My GP, neurologist and the BA doctors have always understood that I will be honest with them. They have trusted me completely to tell them when it is time for me to stop flying. I know now that time isn't far off. But it has to be my decision. If that decision had been made for me, I would have been devastated. BA has given me support, security and understanding and I feel very fortunate that they didn't see the inevitable wheelchair. They are a good example to other companies. I appreciate that not everyone works for a big company and not everyone has a Maggie Sheppard as their manager. Mentally I love my job. Physically, my body hates it.

Having MS has taught me to appreciate how lucky I am. I have met people with chronic progressive MS who have been totally debilitated by their illness and I have stood in admiration at their positive attitude towards their situation. I think that stage would hit me really hard. I fully appreciate what could happen to me. I have to live with that fear every day of my life, but it might never happen. If I spent every moment thinking 'what if ...' I wouldn't be able to get on with my life.

For now, I take each day as it comes and live for today. I have learnt to focus on the things I can do rather than the things I can't. I focus on the good things in my life. It would depend on my circumstances if the worst did happen: where I was living, what job I was doing, whether or not I was single. But to be honest, I rarely think about it. I have become more analytical about life since being diagnosed with MS but sometimes you can analyze things too much. None of us, with MS or not, knows what the future holds. So as my mother has always said: Que sera, sera, what will be, will be ...

I know several people with MS who have chosen to keep it a secret and they have their reasons. Sometimes it can be an easier option, especially in the workplace. I completely understand that as I have been there myself. But for me it was because I didn't want a label. I didn't want people saying: 'You know, that girl with MS.' I'm still me, I'm still Carole Mackie. I didn't want anybody's pity, I just wanted understanding, which I hope this book will achieve for everyone with MS and the people around them.

Also, I think I was afraid to be honest about my MS, mostly because it meant I would have to deal with people's reactions. Again, for me it was facing the not knowing. Not knowing how people would react or how I would deal with their reaction. To be honest, having a secret put me under too much pressure and meant I wasn't receiving the understanding I needed. How could anybody understand what it was like if I didn't tell them how I was feeling? I didn't want to live a lie. It was too much like hard work. Having so much support around me, from BA, my family, friends and colleagues, has given me incredible strength. Without that support, I think things could have been very different.

It's strange, though, writing this book, going public. It means dealing with people's reactions all over again, allowing myself to become public property. Now that is really scary, because I'm not going public just about my MS; it's my thoughts, my feelings, my strengths and my weaknesses. That's what scares me this time. But I know now that it will all be worth it. I am not giving anybody a cure, I am not giving anybody false hope. I am sharing my story with you in the hope that it gives people a better understanding of life with MS. So as someone once said: 'Let's free fall into honesty and hope we survive.'

Appendix

At the end of this appendix there is a list of addresses and telephone numbers where you can obtain further information about all of the treatments and issues mentioned.

WHAT IS MULTIPLE SCLEROSIS?

The name means 'many scars'. The nerve fibres in the brain and spinal cord have a protective sheath called myelin which is a sort of insulation. It helps to conduct electrical impulses between the brain or spinal cord and the rest of the body and prevents them from short-circuiting. When myelin is healthy these electrical impulses get through quickly and accurately and make our movements easy and co-ordinated. When myelin is damaged, or scarred, the messages may be slower, distorted or non-existent.

Symptoms of MS depend on where the myelin is damaged. It can affect the nerves in the brain, the brain stem and spinal cord. Damage to motor nerves affects movement, damage to sensory nerves can alter sensation or cause tingling or numbness. The muscles and organs are not harmed generally, although unused muscles can become spastic; it is simply that the right messages cannot get to and from the brain or through the brain stem and spinal cord.

Multiple sclerosis is not inherited directly. It is neither a contagious nor a fatal disease. For the majority of people with MS, life is not shortened, although young people with MS can expect to live with a lifetime of uncertainty about their disease.

WHO GETS IT?

There are two-and-a-half million people with MS across the world. It is most commonly diagnosed between the ages of 20 and 40. Children can get it, but that is rare. It strikes more women than men. For every three women with MS, two men have it. It is the most common potentially disabling disorder of the nervous system in young adults.

Where you live may affect your chances of developing MS, although nobody knows why. Scotland has the highest incidence anywhere in the world. Roughly two in every thousand of the population have it. In England and Wales, that drops to one in a thousand. In the UK as a whole, 85,000 people have MS. Germany, Iceland, Switzerland and Slovenia have almost as many cases as Scotland.

In America, approximately one third of a million people have MS, mainly in the northern states. It occurs more commonly among people of northern European ancestry, but those of African, Asian and Hispanic backgrounds are not immune. It is also high in Canada and in the southern parts of New Zealand and Australia. In Europe, where the climate grows warmer – Greece, Portugal, Spain – it begins to drop away. MS is almost unknown in tropical countries, although, since health services in these countries are generally busy with epidemic infectious diseases, no one really knows how much less common it is. If you migrate from a cold climate after you are 15, your chances of getting MS stay the same as those of your birthplace.

WHAT CAUSES IT?

No single cause has yet been found. One possible theory is that a virus disturbs the immune system, or indirectly sets off an auto-immune process. In other words, the immune system lets the body's defences turn on themselves. No particular virus has been found to be responsible for MS and some researchers think that a common virus may act as a delayed trigger in genetically susceptible people.

It is thought that some people's genetic make-up may make them more susceptible to MS. Environment may also be involved. MS researchers believe that factors in a child's development up to the age of 15 are important. Many people with MS have had viral illnesses such as chicken pox, measles, flu, herpes, or glandular fever as a child or teenager. Most lived their first 15 years in areas with cold winters.

MS isn't inherited. In the UK, though, the chances of a child having MS when a parent is affected are 20 to 40 times greater than for the general population. That makes the lifetime risk approximately three in every hundred, still much lower than that of developing cancer or heart problems.

WHAT ARE THE SYMPTOMS?

These vary from person to person. It's possible to have different symptoms at different times. Some are very common but there is no typical set of symptoms that apply to everyone. Also, nobody with MS gets ALL the possible symptoms. They can be mild and short-lived or severe and longer-lasting. Some are more common in the early stages of the disease while others occur later. Some may be obvious but others can be invisible, which can be hard to understand for people who don't have MS.

Symptoms may begin with pain at the back of the eyes, double or blurred vision, or nerve pain in the face. Some people have ringing in the ears or hearing problems, tingling, or numbness in the legs, feet, arms and hands. Others get giddiness and loss of balance, muscle weakness, or sudden paralysis of the legs or arms. Some find it difficult to concentrate and become forgetful. Others experience anxiety or depression, or notice other changes in their behaviour.

Fatigue is one of the invisible symptoms which people with MS find difficult to explain to others. MS-related fatigue is different to that experienced by people who don't have MS. It generally occurs on a daily basis, tends to worsen as the day progresses, is often aggravated by heat and humidity, and can come on suddenly and severely. Doctors advise people with MS to manage their stress, sleep and exposure to heat.

Some have speech problems; speech may become slurred or it is difficult to remember a word. Others face problems with bladder or bowel control. Men may find it difficult to get an erection – this can come and go like all other MS symptoms. Both men and women may need more stimulation to stay sexually aroused.

Most single symptoms can be treated or helped. People with MS need to learn what suits them. They can also learn to listen to their body and notice patterns which trigger symptoms. Generally speaking, overexertion, heat, humidity and fever can set off symptoms.

HOW IS MS DIAGNOSED?

It can be difficult to diagnose MS. There is nothing – no single laboratory test, symptom or physical finding – which, when present or positive, always means a person has MS. In addition, some of the symptoms of MS could be caused by other diseases. Therefore a diagnosis of MS must be made carefully, so it can take weeks, months or even years before someone finally learns that they have MS. While waiting for a diagnosis, people often feel frustrated, angry, scared, or start to think that they have become hypochondriacs. 'If the doctor can't tell me what it is, perhaps it's all in my head?'

There is another important factor here: most family doctors will only see two or three cases of people with MS in their entire careers. It is felt that this unfamiliarity with the disease can also delay diagnosis. Doctors usually refer a patient to a neurologist to make or confirm the diagnosis.

Generally speaking, a diagnosis of MS occurs after there have been two sudden worsening of MS symptoms (called 'attacks' or 'exacerbations') within one month and after more than one area of damage to the myelin of the central nervous system has been found.

There are several tests that physicians use to diagnose MS:

Neurological examination   This tests for abnormalities in movement and sensory pathways. The neurologist is looking for changes in eye movements, limb co-ordination, balance, sensation, speech and reflexes, and signs of weakness.

Visual and auditory evoked potentials   Evoked potentials test the time it takes for the brain to receive and interpret messages. Small electrodes are placed on the head to monitor how brain waves respond to stimulation to the eyes and ears. Patients are asked to look at a screen, like a giant black and white board. In a healthy person the response to the images on the screen is almost immediate. If myelin is damaged (known as demyelination) messages take longer to get through.

MRI scan   The MRI (Magnetic Resonance Imaging) scanner is linked to a computer which takes pictures of the brain and spinal cord. It is extremely accurate and can pinpoint the exact place and size of scars on the myelin (also known as plaques or lesions). More than 90 per cent of people with MS have scars that show up on MRI scans. However, some people with MS do not show any myelin damage on a scan.

Lumbar puncture   A needle is inserted into the lower back, under local anaesthetic, and a small sample of the fluid which flows around the brain and spinal cord (cerebrospinal fluid) is taken from the spinal cord. This is then tested for known antibodies.

Other tests   Some conditions mimic MS and these can be ruled out using other tests. These include CT (Computer Axial Tomography) scans, which give an image of a cross-section of the brain; tests to show up certain antibodies in the blood; and inner ear tests to check balance.

WHAT TYPES OF MS ARE THERE?

Multiple sclerosis differs so much from type to type that there is currently debate among scientists and researchers that it could be several different diseases with a common result. People with MS can, therefore, give out conflicting messages. There are four main types of MS, although symptoms and patterns vary within each type from person to person.

Benign MS   This starts with a few mild attacks followed by complete recovery. It doesn't get worse and there is no permanent disability. Around 20 per cent of people with MS have this form. The first symptoms are usually sensory – tingling, burning, pins and needles, numbness.

This form can only be diagnosed when a person has had little or no sign of disability for 10 to 15 years after the first attacks. Sometimes disability will develop after many years of the disease remaining dormant. Some patients have been diagnosed only after they have died and, for other reasons, an autopsy has been carried out on their body.

Relapsing/remitting MS   Seventy per cent of people with MS start with this type. They have attacks (relapses) followed by remissions in which they have fewer, milder or no symptoms.

Relapses tend to be unpredictable and their causes are unknown. During a relapse new symptoms may appear or previous ones will return. A relapse can last for hours, days, weeks or months and vary from mild to severe. At their worst, acute relapses may need hospital treatment.

Remissions are periods of recovery and they can last for years. No one knows what makes the disease go into remission. Even during a remission, myelin damage still shows up on MRI scans.

In the early stages of relapsing/remitting MS, people are often symptom-free during remission. After several attacks, as myelin damage increases, there may be residual damage. The person will then be slightly more affected than before the relapse.

Secondary progressive MS   This starts in the same way as relapsing/remitting MS but after repeated relapses the remissions stop and the MS moves into a progressive phase. Of those who start with relapsing/remitting MS, about 45 per cent go on to this phase. The time span varies. Usually, a person will move into the secondary progressive phase within 15 to 20 years of first diagnosis.

Primary progressive MS   Some people with MS never have relapses and remissions. From the start they experience steadily worsening symptoms and progressive disability. This can level off, or may continue to grow worse. Around 15 per cent of people diagnosed are in this category and this form can shorten life expectancy.

A BRIEF HISTORY

Multiple sclerosis was first described as a distinct disease in 1868. At that time it was blamed on over-exertion. Later it was thought to be caused by infection, poison or a faulty metabolism. Until the early 1900s treatments included laxatives, strychnine, belladonna (medicine from the poisonous deadly nightshade plant), arsenic, iodine and bed rest.

In 1916, James Dawson revealed the basic processes at work with a microscopic description of diseased brain tissue. Treatments then snowballed. Patients had their tonsils removed. They were given psychotherapy, massage, vitamins and special diets. They were given anti-allergy injections, drugs to restrict the flow of blood in their blood vessels – and drugs to increase the flow of blood through their blood vessels. There were no controlled studies carried out and none of the treatments showed any lasting benefits.

In 1946, Sylvia Lawry founded the National MS Society in the United States, the first such society in the world. Two years later research linked MS to the immune system for the first time. The MS Society of Great Britain and Northern Ireland was founded in 1953 and the National Multiple Sclerosis Society of Australia was formed in 1971.

In 1965 criteria for the diagnosis of MS were developed, and during the sixties controlled clinical trials in MS were launched. In 1975 a family susceptibility to MS was first described. The MRI scan first showed pictures of the brain damage caused by MS in 1981. In 1992 an international effort to identify the genes that make people susceptible to MS began.

Three different beta interferon products have been licensed since 1994: Betaferon (beta interferon 1b, branded Betaseron in the US); Avonex (beta interferon 1a); and Rebif (beta interferon 1a)[1]. Avonex and Rebif contain the same ingredients but are manufactured by two different companies which have given the drug different names. In America, the Food and Drug Administration has approved Avonex, Betaseron and a third drug, Copaxone (glatiramer acetate)[2] – commonly called the 'ABC drugs'. These drugs are the first to have a definite positive impact on the disease, and bring hope for further treatments in the near future – and, some day, a cure. They reduce the number of attacks in relapsing/remitting MS, limit the amount of damage in the central nervous system as seen on MRI, and slow down the progression of disability.

In the UK, Avonex and Betaseron are available on the NHS but not all health authorities use them as their cost, at approximately £10,000 per patient per year, is considered prohibitive. It is likely that Betaferon will also be licensed for secondary progressive MS. Copaxone is also being considered by the licensing bodies to reduce the number of attacks in relapsing/remitting MS.

---

1 Betaferon and Avonex are forms of beta interferon, a substance made by the immune system. Rebif is not available in Australia at present.

2 A synthetic which mimics a component of human myelin, perhaps serving as a decoy for the MS attack on myelin.

CURRENT RESEARCH

The aim of research into the causes of MS is, of course, to prevent it happening in the first place. Nobody knows why each person's symptoms vary so greatly or even whether they all stem from the same cause. This is what makes research into the disease so complex. Basically, scientists need to discover how myelin becomes damaged. Only then can they work on ways to limit that damage and encourage repair.

At present there are 60 trials for therapies for MS being carried out around the world. More than half of them are in the United States, where the National MS Society and the National Institutes of Health, a group of federal agencies, provide the vast majority of MS research and training support in every conceivable biomedical research area. The National MS Society has been active in supporting research since 1946 and has allocated over $200 million for research programmes. Because of such support, more is known today than ever before about MS, and this new knowledge is rapidly developing into new strategies for treatment and management of the disease.

Research is taking place on several fronts: geography, the environment in which MS is more common, genetics, diet and micro-organisms. Researchers think a number of micro-organisms could act as a trigger to MS.

To understand how the immune system – normally our first line of defence against infections – might be the source of damage in MS, the scientific and medical community is focusing on research areas essential to the understanding of why and how MS affects the brain and spinal cord. These areas are immunology, genetics, virology and the biology of 'glial' cells – the cells that make and maintain myelin in the central nervous system. These areas of biomedical investigation, interacting together in complex ways, drive current multiple sclerosis research.

Because the cause of MS is unknown, research also focuses on easing symptoms. This includes new methods of reducing tremor and spasticity, alleviating fatigue and evaluating cognitive problems.

Other issues, such as the role of physiotherapy and counselling in the management of MS, are also being researched.

TREATMENTS FOR MS

There is still no known cure for MS. The new drug treatments lessen the frequency or severity of attacks and slow the increase of disability in relapsing-remitting MS. The new drugs may be especially helpful very early in the course of the disease as permanent damage to the underlying nerve fibres occurs early in MS, when outward signs of the disease may be minimal. There are other therapies that can help with individual symptoms:

Physical Therapy (physiotherapy) and Occupational Therapy   Physical therapy can teach a person with MS how to recover good posture, with an emphasis on the right way to stand, to walk, to rise from a sitting or lying position, and the best positions for sleeping.

The benefits can include more normal and easier movement and consequently the chance to enjoy a more active life. MS patients can be shown how to control and co-ordinate movement, reduce spasticity and regain functional abilities.

Exercise programmes, which do not involve raising the body's core temperature, can help strengthen weakened or uncoordinated muscles, keep joints mobile and prevent stiffness, improve co-ordination and balance, boost circulation and prevent pressure sores.

Occupational Therapy (OT) is geared towards improving independence in daily living, by teaching energy conservation methods to combat fatigue, techniques for dressing, grooming, eating and driving and recommending equipment and ways to adapt the home or workplace.

Diet   Good nutrition is essential for everyone, but people with MS may have some special needs when it comes to preparing and eating meals, maintaining proper weight and treating symptoms of MS or other health problems. It is tempting for a person with MS who has continence problems to skip meals and, in particular, to cut down on fluids. But going without food causes weakness and reducing fluids can concentrate the urine which is bad for the kidneys. A healthy diet is important for anyone; for people with MS it can help to fight fatigue and infection.

MS symptoms often reduce mobility of physical activity. If a person is consuming the same amount of calories while activity drops off, the result may be weight gain. The added weight can increase fatigue, further limit mobility and put a strain on the respiratory and circulatory systems. This is the time to pay attention to any calories that provide little nutritional value and to substitute foods that provide more sustained energy. Studies looking at the areas of the world where MS occurs found that it related to the consumption of saturated fats – these are found in dairy products, meat and confectionery. Many people with MS have been advised to follow a low-fat diet.

There are also many nutrition theories or diets that claim to treat MS. These include diets low in gluten, high in polyunsaturated fats, high in certain vitamins, as well as diets which assume that every individual is allergic to certain types of food. Some of these diets are consistent with accepted dietary guidelines and therefore pose no nutritional risk for people with MS. Other diets that claim to be therapeutic may actually work against the principles of proper nutrition. Before considering any 'special' diets, seek information from your MS Society, your doctor or a registered dietician.

Marijuana (Cannabis)   There is on-going debate about the role of marijuana (cannabis) in the treatment of MS, with diverging attitudes in the UK and the US.

Some people with MS claim that smoking marijuana helps to relieve pain and calm muscle spasms, alleviates incontinence and helps them to get a good night's sleep. Others say it does nothing for them at all and a few have reported unpleasant side-effects. These claims led to a small number of clinical trials which explored the role of THC tetrahydrocannabinol (the active ingredient in marijuana) in treating spasticity, tremor and balance control. The studies showed limited results and many side effects. Larger studies are needed to determine if marijuana or its active ingredient is safe and effective in treating MS. In the meantime, there are other, well-tested drugs to help these problems – and marijuana is a controlled substance under the US Drug Enforcement Agency.

The MS Society of Great Britain and Northern Ireland treats marijuana, an illegal drug in the UK, like any potential therapy – it wants

it put under clinical trial. Hundreds of people with MS smoke marijuana or cannabis, as it is more commonly known.

There are hopes that the drug will be licensed as a medicine in the
UK. A clinical trial in which 24 people, most of them with MS, will
be allowed to inhale cannabis begins shortly. They will be exempt
from prosecution for possession of an illegal drug under a special
Home Office licence. As MS is a long-term medical condition which is
very variable, larger and longer trials will also need to take place.

The British Medical Association has added weight to the argument
in favour of legalization. It wants the medicinal properties of the
cannabis plant to be explored. At present it supports the legalization
of cannabinoids, which are molecules derived from the plants.

Cannabis was available on prescription in the UK, in the form of a
tincture, until 1971. It was withdrawn because of its association with
drug abuse. Surveys have shown that doctors are now overwhelm-
ingly in support of being able to prescribe it again.

Alternative and complementary therapies   Each individual with MS
has a unique set of symptoms and a personal way of dealing with
them. Many turn to alternative therapies as a way of easing day-to-
day symptoms, or of raising their general level of health for the fight
against their illness.

These may include homeopathic remedies, aromatherapy, massage,
reflexology – anything which they find effective. Many find that
regular lukewarm baths help to ease muscle tension and fatigue,
aided by the use of aromatherapy oils.

Although it might sound like odd advice, people with MS should
discuss alternative therapies with their doctors. Don't assume that
doctors will automatically reject any alternative; ask your doctor to
explain the risks, benefits, side effects and potential interactions with
medications you are currently taking. Unsupervised therapy can be
dangerous.

FEAR AND ACCEPTANCE

People who are newly-diagnosed can feel shock, anger, fear and grief
when they are told they have MS. Their friends and family may share
some of these emotions. Because the illness usually strikes younger

people they have to come to terms with how MS may change their lives. It is incurable and this often causes profound anger.

A common reaction in the early stages is to deny the illness, or to keep it hidden from other people. Many of the symptoms – fatigue, tingling, burning – are invisible, so this can seem to be the easy way out. But constant denial, on top of coping alone, can become the biggest burden of all. People can become depressed as they face up to their limitations. The fear of other people's reactions to the illness can grow bigger the longer the denial continues. And because the person with MS is keeping the illness hidden, they are not getting the help and support they need. Today, with evidence that early treatment is effective in slowing the onset of long-term consequences, denial is medically ill-advised.

The first big step is accepting the diagnosis. The next step is telling other people. Then it is time to make changes at home and at work to make life easier.

MS Societies advise that counselling or psychotherapy by trained and competent counsellors can help people, particularly in learning to live with the unpredictability of the disease and the grief of losing their health.

STAYING AT WORK WITH MS

Most people are diagnosed with MS when they are in the prime of life so it is tempting to keep the illness a secret from employers. As with friends and family, this can prove more stressful than telling the truth. In the workplace, the fear of being labelled 'That person with MS' can be overwhelming.

Despite the nature of the illness, its unpredictability and its wide range of symptoms, most people will probably be able to hold on to their current jobs. Many people drop out of the work force when they are diagnosed or experience their first major attack. Their decision is made far too quickly. Those who need some time away from work should first investigate sick leave policy, short term disability insurance or even leave without pay. It is almost always easier to return to work than to find a new job.

If someone is having difficulty working to their fullest potential, they should discuss possible accommodations with their employer. In

Britain, the Disability Discrimination Act requires employers to take reasonable measures to ensure they are not discriminating against disabled people. This includes recruitment, training, promotion and dismissal. Big organizations, with their own medical staff, may be able to absorb any problems an employee with MS has. Small companies may not be equipped to deal with it, and those with fewer than 15 employees are exempt from the Act. Not all employers will be sympathetic, either.

In the US, the right to 'reasonable accommodations' is legally provided by the Americans with Disabilities Act (ADA), a civil rights law for people with disabilities. Reasonable accommodations can included adjustments such as flex time, accessible office space, parking privileges or computer software that enhances work performance.

In Australia, the rights of citizens in respect of employment are protected by several Acts – chief amongst which are the Equal Opportunity Act (Vic.) 1995, the Disability Discrimination Act (Cth.) 1992, the Industrial Relations Act with amendments (1994) and the Workplace Relations Act (Cth) 1996

Before requesting any accommodations, an employee should seek information and advice from an occupational therapist, career counsellor or the MS Society. Staff at MS centres have developed specialist knowledge that can help people with MS assess and make informed decisions about their employment, superannuation and legal options.

The nature of the illness, its unpredictability and its wide range of symptoms will make some jobs and professions untenable. Again, big organizations may be able to retrain a person to move to another department, or work out jobshare, flex time and home-working alternatives.

MS can also be a barrier to trying for a new job. Unless it is relevant, no one is required to declare their diagnosis unless asked directly. Deciding whether or not to disclose can be a difficult decision; employees can claim to be discriminated against only if they have declared their diagnosis.

It is wise not to make any hasty decisions, especially when newly-diagnosed and coming to terms with the illness. For some people with MS, the correct decision will be to leave work eventually and use their energy to build an independent and full life outside the workplace.

There are booklets which explain MS to employers and which give details of grants available if the employer needs to adapt the workplace. The emphasis is on the benefits of keeping a known and trusted employee within a company, rather than the need to recruit and train a replacement.

MS AND RELATIONSHIPS

Friends   It is important for people with MS to build and maintain a strong circle of good friends, particularly if they are single. A relapse, or even just a bad day, can strike when the refrigerator is empty or when they've promised to help someone out. They may need their shopping done for them, but they will be equally distraught at letting down a friend and breaking a promise. This can be dealt with through educating friends so that they understand the nature of the disease.

It is also important that friends don't tiptoe around the person with MS. Ordinary life goes on and other people fall ill, have crises or need a shoulder to cry on, too. Not everything should revolve around MS. A person with MS may find that there is a natural 'pruning' and new growth of friendships in the years following diagnosis as needs and lifestyles change. But this is all dependent on the type of MS which is diagnosed and the personality and circumstances of the person with MS.

Family   Family, like friends, will need to be educated in what MS is and how symptoms or relapses affect the person diagnosed with it. Family members will vary in their reactions to the news that someone they love has MS.

They may go into denial and not want to know about the illness or they may want to cosset the 'patient' and attempt to take away some of their independence. After diagnosis, there will be a period of adjustment for everyone that may take some years to resolve.

There can also be jealousy towards the person with MS; they are suddenly the focus of everybody's attention and concern, and will inevitably take up more time than a healthy person.

Family members will experience many of the emotions a newly-diagnosed person has, but from a different perspective. They will worry about what to do during a relapse, or whether the person they have known and loved will change. They may also worry about the long-term consequences: what sort of care and support will be expected of them?

In general, as in the workplace, it is best not to do anything hastily but wait to see what form the MS takes. It is vital to nurture good communication on the subject with close family members as this will take away some of their fears.

Finding a partner, keeping a partner   The fear of the MS growing worse is often greater than the condition itself. If someone whose partner has always been healthy is suddenly diagnosed with an incurable disease it can alter the relationship dramatically. Partners may want to distance themselves from the illness, or even leave. Not everyone can cope in these situations. On the other hand, MS can become a common enemy which creates an even closer bond between couples.

Single people face a different set of issues: when should they tell a date that they have MS? Will they ever meet anyone prepared to take them on? Does it make them less attractive? But people with MS say it also alters what they are looking for in a partner. Communication becomes even more important as the person with MS will need to feel confident that their symptoms – invisible or not – will be understood.

Relationships are put under a particular kind of stress if the person with MS is suffering cognitive problems. Sometimes – although this is rare – the wrong messages will go to the brain and lead to inappropriate behaviour. For example, an MS person may suddenly laugh out loud at a funeral, upsetting other mourners. They may say cruel or hurtful things to those nearest to them and be labelled by others as self-centred or uncaring.

It puts an unbearable strain on a relationship if the person with MS is seen as inconsiderate, selfish or crazy rather than as someone with a genuine medical problem. MS can sometimes lead to difficulties in memory, concentration, self-control and emotional expression; all these symptoms can cause enormous distress, hurt and anger among carers, partners, family and friends.

MS symptoms can also be abused by the person with MS. Fatigue, probably the most difficult symptom to explain, can be used to manipulate a partner. The person with MS can then become a full-time 'invalid', keeping their partner at their beck and call at all times. When one partner has MS, important issues about roles, independence and dependence need to be sorted out – both for the person with MS *and* for the partner. It can also be difficult to switch from the roles of carer/patient to lovers.

Some couples in which one partner has MS choose to have all caring or nursing tasks carried out by professionals or non-family members so that their core relationship is not affected. This can be very expensive and is not always possible, however.

SEX

There has been very little research into sexual problems associated with MS but recent evidence suggests that around 75 per cent, or three-quarters, of people with MS experience some sexually-related problems at some time. However, the rate of sexual problems in the general population is also very high, and like most other symptoms, these come and go. Some sexual difficulties are caused by changes in the central nervous system due to MS, while others may be the result of the emotional and social consequences of living with MS.

The main problems reported by women with MS are fatigue, decreased or altered sensation, poor lubrication, lack of sexual interest or drive (more common among women with MS than men), difficulty with arousal and lack of orgasm.

The most common problem among men with MS is getting or maintaining an erection. Premature or retarded ejaculation, loss of sexual interest or desire, decreased frequency of masturbation and fatigue are also common.

If the person with MS has incontinence problems, it can create so much anxiety that sex is neglected. Similarly, it can be difficult for a person to think of themselves as sexually desirable if they have to be lifted from a wheelchair onto the bed. These are the sort of problems which can drive a wedge between couples. Help is available but again, it can take courage to seek it on such intimate matters.

Couples may find they have to bring up the subject of sex-related problems with their doctor, although some may be reluctant to discuss such matters, seeing it as an intrusion of privacy.

HAVING CHILDREN

MS has no effect on female fertility so if a woman with MS wants to have a child, MS generally won't prevent it. Studies have confirmed that pregnant women have fewer attacks during pregnancy. Some researchers think pregnancy hormones suppress the immune system, decreasing the activity of the disease. Pregnancy, delivery and breastfeeding can be the same as for mothers who do not have MS.

The first six months after childbirth, however, present a greater risk. A European study of mothers with MS has shown a 30 per cent increase in attacks during this time. After this time, the rate of attack returns to the levels it was at before pregnancy. Even without MS, babies and young children are tiring and a mother with MS may need people to help her so that her new lifestyle doesn't make her too fatigued.

Men with MS can become fathers. If there are problems with impotence, these can be overcome by locally injecting a drug which gives an erection or by using a vacuum pump. Viagra may also help men with MS. Unlike other products, this drug is taken orally and does not give an erection automatically, just in response to sexual stimulation.

Address Book

Here are some telephone numbers, addresses and websites where you can get information, leaflets and help on any aspect of MS and MS-related issues in Great Britain and Northern Ireland, the Irish Republic, the United States and Australia. For addresses of other MS Societies, contact:

The International Federation of Multiple Sclerosis Societies
10 Heddon Street
London WIR 7LJ
England
Tel: (44) 171 734 9120
Fax: (44) 171 287 2587
e-mail: info@ifmss.org.uk

(*in England*)
The Multiple Sclerosis Society
25 Effie Road
Fulham
London SW6 1EE
Tel: 0171 610 7171
Fax: 0171 736 9861
e-mail: info@mssociety.org.uk

(*in Scotland*)
The Multiple Sclerosis Society
2a North Charlotte Street
Edinburgh EH2 4HR
Tel: 0131 225 3600
Fax: 0131 220 5188

(*in Northern Ireland*)
The Multiple Sclerosis Society
34 Annadale Avenue
Belfast BT7 3JJ
Tel: 01232 802802
Fax: 01232 802803

(*in the Irish Republic*)
The Multiple Sclerosis Society
2 Sandymount Green
Dublin 4
Tel: (353 1) 269 4599
Fax: (353 1) 269 3746
e-mail: mssoi@iol.ie

MS Helpline
0171 371 8000
(Open Monday-Friday, 10 a.m.-4 p.m. and some evenings)
This offers support, help and information for anyone with MS, their family, partner or friends.

MS Telephone Counselling Service
London: 0171 222 3123 (24 hours)
Midlands: 0121 476 4229
Scotland: 0131 226 6573

Multiple Sclerosis Resource Centre
4a Chapel Hill
Stansted
Essex CM24 8AG
Tel: 01279 817101
Fax: 01279 647179
Information helpline, book list, training, advice, and a quarterly magazine.

The British Homoeopathic Association
27a Devonshire Street
London W1N 1RJ
Tel: 0171 935 2163
The Association can supply a list of registered homeopaths in your area.

Carersline Helpline
Tel: 0345 573369
(Monday-Friday, 10 a.m.-midday, 2 p.m.-4 p.m.)

Carers National Association
Ruth Pitter House
20-25 Glasshouse Yard
London EC1A 4JS
Tel: 0171 490 8818
Fax: 0171 490 8824

The Continence Foundation
307 Hatton Square
16 Baldwin's Garden
London EC1N 7RJ
Tel: 0171 404 6875
Fax: 0171 404 6876

Disabled Drivers Association
National Headquarters
Ashwellthorpe
Norwich NR16 1EX
Tel: 01508 489449
Fax: 01508 488173

The Federation of MS Therapy Centres
Bradbury House
155 Barkers Lane
Bedford MK41 9RX
Tel: 01234 325781
Fax: 01234 365242

Motability
Goodman House
Station Approach
Harlow
Essex CM20 2ET
Tel: 01279 635666
Fax: 01279 632000

Natural Medicines Society
Market Chambers
13a Market Place
Heanor
Derbyshire DE75 7AA
Tel: 01773 710002
Fax: 01858 469373

The Pain Society
9 Bedford Square
London WC1B 3RA
Tel: 0171 636 2750
Fax: 0171 323 2015
For advice on self-help pain management for those with chronic, persistent pain.

SPOD
(Association to Aid the Sexual and Personal Relationships of People with a Disability)
286 Camden Road
London N7 OBJ
Tel: 0171 607 8851

Yoga for Health Foundation
Ickwell Bury
Nr Biggleswade
Bedfordshire SG18 9EF
Tel: 01767 627271
Fax: 01767 627266
Produces a tape called *Yoga And Multiple Sclerosis*, runs residential courses for people with MS.

United States

The National MS Society
733 Third Avenue
New York
NY 10017
Tel: Call 1-800-FIGHT MS (1-899-344-4867) and select option #1 to be connected with the chapter nearest you.
e-mail: info@nmss.org
Your local chapter will also be listed in the Yellow Pages under 'Multiple Sclerosis'.

Australia

National Multiple Sclerosis Society of Australia
34 Jackson Street
Toorak VIC 3142
Australia
Tel: 03 9828 7222
Fax: 03 9826 9054
e-mail: public@mssociety.com.au

Australian Capital Territory
Gloria McKerrow House
117 Denison Street
Deakin ACT 2600
Tel: 02 6285 2999
Fax: 02 6281 0817

New South Wales
Level 11, 447 Kent Street
Sydney NSW 2000
Tel: 02 9287 2929
Fax: 02 9287 2987
e-mail: msnsw@msnsw.org.au
Information Line: 1800 042 138

Queensland
286 Gladstone Road
Dutton Park QLD 4102
Tel: 07 3840 0888
Fax: 07 3840 0813
e-mail: mssociety@ms-qld.aust.com
Information Line: 1800 177 591

South Australia
274 North East Road
Klemzig SA 5087
Tel: 08 8266 2311
Fax: 08 8266 3522
e-mail: network@ms.asn.au
Information Line: 1800 812 311

Tasmania
15 Princes Street
Sandy Bay TAS 7005
Tel: 03 6224 4111
Fax: 03 6224 4222
Information Line: 1800 676 721

Victoria
See National Multiple Sclerosis Society of Australia
Information line: 1800 816 113

Western Australia
29 Parkhill Way
Wilson WA 6107
Tel: 08 9365 4846
Fax: 08 9451 4453
e-mail: multiple@multiple-wa.asn.au

Address correspondence to Multiple Sclerosis Society of (appropriate region)

ADDRESSES OF OTHER
USEFUL ORGANIZATIONS:

Continence Foundation of Australia
Park Street
Parkville VIC 3052
Tel: 03 9388 8033

Association for the Blind Vision Resource Centre
454 Glenferrie Road
Kooyong VIC 3144
Tel: 03 9822 1111
Fax: 03 9864 9210

Independent Living Centre
705 Geelong Road
Brooklyn VIC 3012
Tel: 30 9362 6111

Websites

The Multiple Sclerosis Society of Great Britain and Northern Ireland
http://www.mssociety.org.uk

The National MS Society (US)
http://www.nmss.org

International Federation of MS Societies: The World of MS
http://www.ifmss.org.uk

Jooly's Joint
(A free worldwide webpal site set up by Julie Howell, who has MS)
http://www.mswebpals.org

Medline
(Medical information service, useful for up-to-date reports on research into MS. Abstracts are free but there is a charge for full texts of online medical journals)
http://www.healthworks.co.uk

AUSTRALIAN WEBSITES

On health issues in general:
http://www.health.gov.au/hfs
Australian Department of Health and Family Services

http://www.dgcs.gov.au/
Department of Family and Community Services

http://www.dircsa.org.au/
Disability Information and Resource Centre SA

http://www.disabilityinfo.org.au/
Disability Information Victoria
Information Line: 1300 650 865

http://www.ms.asn.au/society
MS Society of South Australia

On carers and caregiving:
http://www.carers.asn.au/
Carers Association of Australia

On employment issues and disability:
http://www.vicnet.net.au/vicnet/co mmunity/deac.html
Disability Employment Action Centre Inc.